Tumor
Imaging

Tumor Imaging
Current State of the Art and Recommendations for Future Research

David G. Bragg, M.D.
Professor and Chairman
Department of Radiology
University of Utah School of Medicine
and Medical Center
Salt Lake City, Utah

William R. Hendee, Ph.D.
Professor and Chairman
Department of Radiology
University of Colorado School of Medicine
Denver, Colorado

APPLETON-CENTURY-CROFTS/Norwalk, Connecticut

82 83 84 85 86 / 10 9 8 7 6 5 4 3 2 1

Prentice-Hall International, Inc., London
Prentice-Hall of Australia, Pty. Ltd., Sydney
Prentice-Hall of India Private Limited, New Delhi
Prentice-Hall of Japan, Inc., Tokyo
Prentice-Hall of Southeast Asia (Pte.) Ltd., Singapore
Whitehall Books Ltd., Wellington, New Zealand

Library of Congress Cataloging in Publication Data
Main entry under title:

Tumor imaging.

   Includes bibliographies and index.
   Contents: New imaging technologies in oncologic
diagnosis / William R. Hendee—X-ray transmission
computed tomography / William R. Hendee—Ultrasound /
Marc S. Lapayowker, Marvin C. Ziskin, and Richard A.
Banjavic—[etc.]
   1. Cancer—Diagnosis. 2. Radiography, Medical.
3. Imaging systems in medicine. I. Bragg, David G.
II. Hendee, William R., 1938–
RC270.T858   616.99'40757   82-6725
ISBN 0-8385-9042-X   A9042-1

Cover and text design: Gloria J. Moyer
Production Editor: Gerard G. East

PRINTED IN THE UNITED STATES OF AMERICA

Contributors

Robert Anderson, M.D.
Professor of Radiology
University of Utah School of
   Medicine and Medical Center
Salt Lake City, Utah

Richard A. Banjavic, Ph.D.
Assistant Professor of Radiology
Department of Radiology
University of Colorado School of
   Medicine
Denver, Colorado

David G. Bragg, M.D.
Professor and Chairman
University of Utah School of
   Medicine and Medical Center
Salt Lake City, Utah

Ronald A. Castellino, M.D.
Associate Professor of Radiology
Stanford University
Stanford, California

Gerald D. Dodd, M.D.
Professor and Head
Department of Diagnostic Radiology
University of Texas
M.D. Anderson Hospital and Tumor
   Institute
Houston, Texas

Leonard M. Freeman, M.D.
Professor of Radiology, Co-Director,
   Division of Nuclear Medicine
Department of Radiology
Albert Einstein Medical College
Bronx, New York

Alexander Gottschalk, M.D.
Professor of Diagnostic Radiology
Department of Radiology
Yale University School of Medicine
New Haven, Connecticut

Herman Grossman, M.D.
Professor of Radiology and Pediatrics
Duke University Medical Center
Durham, North Carolina

William R. Hendee, Ph.D.
Professor and Chairman
Department of Radiology
University of Colorado School of
   Medicine
Denver, Colorado

Paul B. Hoffer, M.D.
Professor of Diagnostic Radiology,
   Director, Section of Nuclear
   Medicine
Department of Radiology
Yale University School of Medicine
New Haven, Connecticut

Christopher C. Kuni, M.D.
Assistant Professor of Radiology
Department of Radiology
Division of Nuclear Medicine
University of Colorado School of
   Medicine
Denver, Colorado

Marc S. Lapayowker, M.D.
Professor of Radiology
Temple University Hospital
Philadelphia, Pennsylvania

Gwilym S. Lodwick, M.D.
Professor of Radiology
University of Missouri School of
   Medicine
Columbus, Ohio

John R. Milbrath, M.D.
Associate Professor of Radiology
The Medical College of Wisconsin
Milwaukee, Wisconsin

Franklin J. Miller, M.D.
Associate Professor, Director,
   Vascular Radiology
Department of Radiology
University of Utah School of
   Medicine and Medical Center
Salt Lake City, Utah

Anthony V. Proto, M.D.
Associate Professor of Radiology
University of Cincinnati College of
  Medicine
Cincinnati, Ohio

Lee F. Rogers, M.D.
Professor and Chairman
Department of Radiology
Northwestern University School of
  Medicine
Chicago, Illinois

Carol M. Rumack, M.D.
Assistant Professor of Radiology
University of Colorado School of
  Medicine
Denver, Colorado

Barry Siegel, M.D.
Professor of Radiology, Director,
  Division of Nuclear Medicine
Department of Radiology
Mallinckrodt Institute of Radiology
St. Louis, Missouri

Garry D. Strauser
Assistant Professor of Radiology,
  Chief, Uroradiology Section
Department of Radiology
University of Colorado School of
  Medicine
Denver, Colorado

William Strauss, M.D.
Assistant Radiologist, Director,
  Division of Nuclear Medicine
Massachusetts General Hospital
Boston, Massachusetts

Jerome F. Wiot, M.D.
Professor and Chairman
Department of Radiology
University of Cincinnati College of
  Medicine
Cincinnati, Ohio

Charles R. Wilson, Ph.D.
Associate Professor of Radiology
The Medical College of Wisconsin
Milwaukee, Wisconsin

James E. Youker, M.D.
Professor and Chairman
Department of Radiology
The Medical College of Wisconsin
Milwaukee, Wisconsin

Bernard E. Zeligman, M.D.
Instructor in Radiology
Department of Radiology
University of Colorado School of
  Medicine
Denver, Colorado

Marvin C. Ziskin, M.D.
Professor of Radiology and Medical
  Physics
Department of Radiology
Temple University Medical School
Philadelphia, Pennsylvania

Contents

Preface

The imaging of tumors by radiologic methods has been neither recognized as a separate discipline of radiology nor integrated effectively into the organizational matrix of most services of clinical radiology. As a result, the clinical and research accomplishments of this specialty area of radiology have been compromised, and the delineation of tumor imaging as a unified subject involving all aspects of radiologic imaging has been neglected. Identification of tumor imaging as a viable enterprise within the field of radiologic imaging is the purpose of this book.

The book is comprised of a series of position papers covering the discipline of tumor imaging. Some of the papers are oriented towards imaging disciplines, while others are directed towards specific anatomical regions where tumor imaging is important. The papers are presented in a standard format that includes a state-of-the-art description of the imaging area and an outline of specific areas needing additional support for research. The areas of research support are assigned rankings with respect to priority and probability for success and include an estimated timetable for completion.

In the papers of this volume, certain areas of redundancy occur. For example, emission computed tomography is discussed in the chapters on "New Imaging Technologies in Oncologic Diagnosis" and "Nuclear Medicine." Similarly, certain interventional angiographic techniques are described in the chapter on angiography as well as in the chapters on gastrointestinal radiology and head and neck radiology. These occasional areas of overlap are important enough to warrant discussion in more than one location in the book.

The chapters in this book are an outgrowth of the Strategic Plan in Radiologic Sciences for the National Cancer Program-Imaging Subcommittee, which was formed in 1977 under the Commission on Cancer of the American College of Radiology. Financial support for the Subcommittee's efforts was derived in part from contract number CA 25791 from the National Cancer Institute. The Imaging Subcommittee has developed a series of recommendations proclaiming the need for increased support of tumor imaging. Among the recommendations are:

1. An oncologic imaging advisory committee to the National Cancer Institute should be established to make available a spectrum of individuals with specific imaging expertise. By this process, experts in tumor imaging would be available to the various oncologic groups responsible for developing and monitoring diagnostic, treatment, and research protocols, grants, and contracts.

2. The emerging subspecialty field of diagnostic oncologic imaging (di-

agnostic oncoradiology) needs both enhanced visibility and increased financial support. Training funds and committee representation within the National Cancer Institute would facilitate the emergence of this discipline in training institutions across the country. These efforts have the potential for improving the coordination and application of oncologic imaging procedures in training institutions and, subsequently, the community of practicing physicians.

3. At the technical and professional levels, the standardization of radiologic procedures as they relate to tumor imaging needs improvement. Educational efforts should be focused on the efficacious application of imaging studies in the diagnosis, workup, and follow-up of cancer patients.

As the field of tumor imaging gains increased recognition within the field of radiology, advances are anticipated which may change the character of this imaging discipline. To accommodate these changes, the present volume has been prepared in a soft-cover format which is adaptable to periodic updating and revision. The authors intend to provide these updates and revisions so that the text will remain as dynamic as the field itself.

David G. Bragg, M.D.
William R. Hendee, Ph.D.

ONE

New Imaging Technologies in Oncologic Diagnosis

William R. Hendee

INTRODUCTION AND BACKGROUND

Essential to continued improvement in the detection and delineation of cancer by radiologic imaging techniques is the evolution of new imaging methods for acquiring anatomic and physiologic information about the patient. As these methods evolve to the status of proven reliability, they are incorporated into the clinical armamentarium of the radiologist and become part of the set of procedures which he has available to identify pathologic processes which may be present within the patient. Among more recent examples of the evolution of new imaging technologies to the status of proven reliability are neurologic applications of computed tomography, rare-earth screen film combinations and their applications to a variety of roentgenographic imaging procedures, including mammography, and gray-scale display of ultrasound B-mode images.

At any given moment, as certain new imaging technologies are finding applications in the clinical arena, others are in various stages of design or development. In most cases, those technologies with high potential for useful clinical applications in radiology would evolve eventually into the clinical arena without the assistance of external influences. On the other hand, this evolution can be expedited by judicious allocation of financial and manpower resources focused upon selected technologies with high potential for clinical utility. This focusing of resources requires a constant

Gratitude is expressed to Dr. Gordon Brownell, Massachusetts General Hospital, for review of and additions to this chapter.

1

effort to identify promising imaging technologies early in their development. Such identification is the subject of this report.

In the identification of promising imaging technologies, a continuous, objective appraisal of the scientific merit of various imaging developments is essential if financial and manpower resources are to be employed most efficiently. For this purpose, any agency with responsibility for employment of these resources should solicit and follow the advice of volunteer advisory committees composed of individuals with expertise in imaging technology. Responsibilities of these committees should include the design of comparative and correlative studies among various imaging modalities and the development of evaluation protocols to ensure that comparative and correlative studies are not influenced by subjective preference of designers of the studies for one modality over another. In addition, the advisory committees should monitor the allocation of personnel and financial resources to guard against the reorientation of resources to new projects to the detriment of promising projects already receiving support.

RECOMMENDATIONS FOR RESEARCH SUPPORT

At the present time, at least four emerging imaging technologies appear promising as potentially useful clinical techniques for the detection and delineation of cancer (Table 1-1). These technologies are: (1) nuclear magnetic resonance imaging, also known as zeugmatography; (2) microwave thermographic imaging; (3) ultrasound computed tomography; and (4) emission computed tomography. The principles, potential applications, and limitations of each of these technologies are discussed below.

Nuclear Magnetic Resonance Imaging

In this imaging technique, the patient is placed inside a ring-shaped magnet which furnishes a static magnetic field.[1-3] A transmitter inside the magnet emits radiofrequency pulses at a right angle to the static magnetic field. During the quiescent period between pulses, a pick-up coil inside the ring magnet detects radiofrequency signals from the sampling volume. These signals reflect proton densities as well as spin-lattice and spin-spin relaxation times of nuclei within the sampling volume. The signals are translated into a gray-scale image on a television display as the sampling volume is scanned through a cross-sectional slice within the patient.[4,5] The gray-scale image can be used to portray the anatomy of the cross-sectional volume, as shown in Figure 1-1. In such an image, tissues are distinguished by characteristic nuclear relaxation times which may in part reflect differences in the structure and amount of intracellular water. In

TABLE 1-1. SUMMARY OF RESEARCH RECOMMENDATIONS FOR TUMOR IMAGING WITH NEW IMAGING TECHNOLOGIES

Project	Priority	Duration (yr)	Probability of Success
Nuclear magnetic resonance imaging	1	5	Moderate
Microwave thermography	1	3	Moderate
Ultrasound computed tomography	1	5	Excellent
Emission computed tomography	2	5	Low–moderate for cancer detection

some instances, normal and neoplastic tissues differ in intracellular water content, and this difference has been proposed as a mechanism for cancer detection by zeugmatography.[6-10]

Nuclear magnetic resonance imaging and tumor detection are in a rather primitive state of development at this time, and the potential of this technology for clinical utilization is difficult to assess. Although no deleterious biologic effects are expected for this imaging modality, the complexity and expense of the technique are anticipated limitations. Nevertheless, nuclear magnetic resonance imaging should be pursued as one of the technologies to receive a focused allocation of funding resources.

Priority: 1
Duration: 5 years
Probability of Success: moderate for cancer detection

Microwave Thermographic Imaging
The usefulness of infrared thermography for detection of tumors in any anatomic region, including the breast, is severely limited by the rapid absorption of infrared radiation in tissue. This rapid absorption allows detection of only the radiation originating within very superficial layers of tissue. For this reason, infrared thermographic images are confined essentially to display of temperature profiles of the skin surface. Although these profiles may indicate the presence of thermal abnormalities related to the neoplasms, inflammations, and circulatory disturbances below the skin surface, the reliability of this relationship is unsatisfactory because of anomalies in the superficial heat pattern introduced by ambiguous transfer of the underlying heat pattern to the surface.

One approach to improving the correlation between the thermographic data and deep-seated thermal abnormalities is detection and quantitative

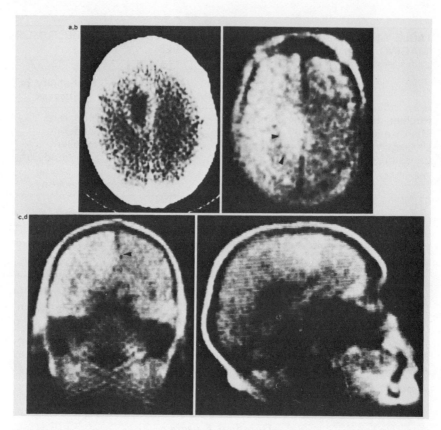

FIGURE 1-1. Right parasagittal posterior frontal glioma in a 54-year-old man who presented with a progressive left hemiparesis. **A:** Postcontrast axial transverse CT scan shows the tumor as an area of low attenuation surrounded by a peripheral dense rim. **B:** Axial transverse NMR scan is of a comparable section and shows tumor to be a homogeneous area of high density with ill-defined margins *(arrowheads).* **C:** Coronal NMR scan shows extension of the tumor to the medial surface of the hemisphere with compression and partial obliteration of the inter-hemispheric fissure *(arrowhead).* **D:** Right parasagittal scan shows the downward extension of tumor into the body of the lateral ventricle. *(From Hawkes RC, et al: J Comput Assist Tomogr 4:577–586, 1980)*

or visual display of longer-wavelength, more penetrating radiation emanating naturally from the body. Suitable radiation has a wavelength on the order of millimeters or centimeters rather than the micrometer wavelength radiation employed for infrared thermography, and quantitative data and images formed with this radiation depict thermal abnormalities from deeper regions of the body. For example, a penetration depth of 2 cm is provided by 2.4 GHz radiation in tissue.[11,12] However, the greater penetration of longer wavelength radiation is accompanied by a reduction in spatial resolution, and judgment is required in selecting an imaging frequency appropriate to the anatomic region of interest. For detection of breast cancer, preliminary results indicate that this frequency is on the order of 20 to 30 GHz.[13,14]

Medical applications of long-wavelength thermography include imaging of the breast for detection of breast cancer and imaging of joints for evaluation of the effectiveness of treatment for arthritis and other inflammatory conditions. A 30 GHz mm-wavelength image of a patient with suspected breast cancer is shown in Figure 1-2.

Long-wavelength thermographic studies are being conducted at the Massachusetts Institute of Technology,[15] at the University of Colorado Health Sciences Center,[16] and possibly also at other institutions. Funding for these investigations is rather meager, and a higher investment of resources conceivably might lead to a more rapid assessment of the clinical utility of this technique. For this reason, some additional focusing of resources on long-wavelength thermography is recommended.

Priority: 1
Duration: 3 years
Probability of Success: Moderate for cancer detection

Ultrasound Computed Tomography

In the imaging technique known as ultrasound computed tomography, focused transmitting and receiving transducers on opposite sides of the patient move in synchrony through a combination of translational and rotational motions. These motions are similar to those employed for first generation x-ray computed tomographic units. In one mode of operation, measurements of ultrasound transmission at increments throughout the scanning process are subjected to an image reconstruction algorithm to provide cross-sectional images of ultrasound attenuation similar to attenuation images furnished in x-ray computed tomography.[17,18] In another mode of operation, measurements are obtained of the time of flight of ultrasound pulses at increments across the scanning motion, and from these measurements a cross-sectional image is reconstructed of ultrasound velocity across the region of interest.[19-21]

To date, most of the experimental work involving ultrasound computed tomography has been directed towards breast imaging, with the breast suspended in a water medium maintained at a temperature which provides an ultrasound velocity matching the average velocity of ultrasound in the breast. Shown in Figure 1-3 are attentuation (left) and velocity (right) images of the breast of a patient with some fibrocystic develop-

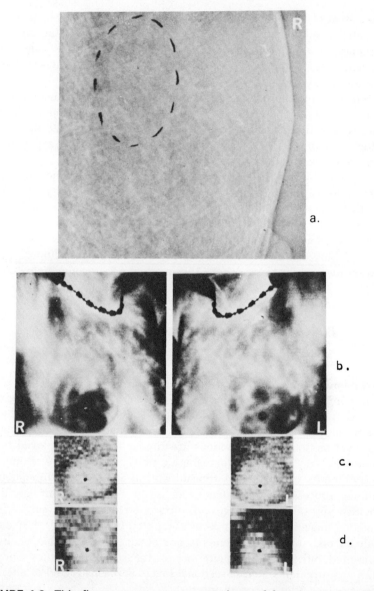

FIGURE 1-2. This figure presents a comparison of four breast imaging modalities. **A:** A xeroradiograph of the right breast of a patient with cystic pathology. **B:** A conventional infrared thermogram of the same patient showing a slight increase in temperature in the caudal region of the right breast. **C, D:** Mm-wavelength thermograms (λ = 0.4 cm and 1.0 cm, respectively) demonstrating elevated temperatures in the right breast.

ment. These images were obtained with 19 mm diameter, 3.5 MHz ultrasound transducers. It is anticipated that conventional B-mode pulse echo images will be obtainable simultaneously with attenuation and velocity images. Also, cross-sectional velocity data are transformable into indices of refraction which may be useful in correcting pulse echo B-mode images for distortion due to refraction. Similar techniques may be applicable to determination of the temperature distribution in tissues subjected to hyperthermic procedures during cancer therapy.

Although limited to relatively homogeneous tissues without large gradients in acoustic impedance, ultrasound computed tomography is a promising imaging technique for such tissues as the breast. The technique is being pursued by researchers at General Electric Company, the Mayo Clinic, and the University of Colorado Health Sciences Center. More rapid progress would be achievable with an increased allotment of man-

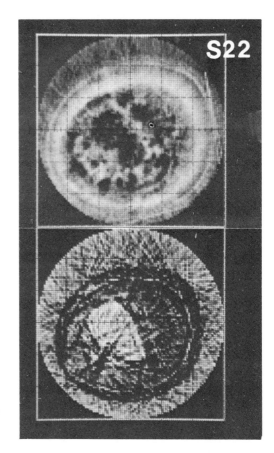

FIGURE 1-3. Attenuation *(left)* and the velocity *(right)* images of the breast of a patient with a 3 cm cyst. The images were obtained with 19 mm diameter 3.5 MHz transducer.

power and support resources, and for this reason increased emphasis on the technique is encouraged.

Priority: 1
Duration: 5 years
Probability of Success: 0.7—high for cancer detection

Emission Computed Tomography

A number of investigators have explored various approaches to computed tomographic imaging of the distribution of gamma-emitting radionuclides in the body. Perhaps the most promising application of this technique is coincidence imaging of the positron-emitting nuclides C-11, N-13, and O-15. The short half-life of these nuclides requires that the imaging facility and a cyclotron for production of the radionuclides be in close proximity. This requirement necessitates a rather expensive facility for computed tomographic imaging with C-11, N-13, and O-15. Advantages include the feasibility of isotopic labeling of a variety of compounds with these nuclides and the availability of annihilation radiation for coincidence counting, a technique which reduces a number of difficulties associated with computed tomographic imaging of conventional gamma-emitting nuclides.[22] Other potential applications of positron emission computed tomography involve the positron emitting radionuclides Flourine-18 (F-18) and gallium-68 (Ga-68), which may be produced in a generator by decay of germanium-68 (Ge-68).

Among the applications of emission computed tomography presently being explored with both single and annihilation photon imaging techniques are cardiac imaging, brain studies involving determination of blood flow and oxygen utilization, and detection of pulmonary emboli.[23-26] Although applications of emission computed tomography to cancer detection are rather speculative, studies should be conducted to assess the potential of this technique to identify tumors based upon physiologic criteria measured tomographically. These studies should be encouraged, and their support by judicious allocation of resources would seem justifiable.

Priority: 2
Duration: 5 years
Probability of Success: low for cancer detection

With the advent of new imaging technologies exemplified by the methods described above, opportunities are promising for the development of innovative quantitative methods for tissue characterization and detection of cancer and for the identification of techniques to follow tissue changes during a course of therapy (Table 1-1). For example, perturbations in reflected and transmitted ultrasound pulses are introduced by the medium traversed by the pulses, and these perturbations or "signatures" should be susceptible to interpretation in terms of the composition of the medium. At Case Western Reserve University, the absorption of 10 GHz microwave radiation in fat and muscle is being investigated as a preliminary feasibility study of microwave computed tomography for detection of soft tissue tumors. At a number of institutions, studies are under way of the utilization of quantitative transmission computed tomographic data for characterization of tissues and identification of tumors. Similar studies are in progress at a few institutions for evaluation of the contribution of emission computed tomography to tissue characterization and quantitative physiology. To exploit the potential of these investigative approaches, correlative tissue characterization studies are needed which employ a variety of imaging modalities, such as ultrasound, microwave thermography, zeugmatography, and emission and transmission computed tomography. Allocation of manpower and financial resources in support of such studies is strongly recommended.

REFERENCES

1. Lauterbur PC: Image formation by induced local interaction: Examples employing nuclear magnetic resonance. Nature 242:190, 1973.
2. Mansfield P: Multi-planar image formation using NMR spin echoes. J Phys [C] 10:L55, 1977.
3. Mansfield P, Maudsley AA: Medical imaging by NMR. Br J Radiol 50:188, 1977.
4. Lauterbur PC, Kramer DM, House WV, Chem C: Zeugmatographic high resolution nuclear magnetic resonance spectroscopy: Images of chemical inhomogeneity within macroscopic objects. J Am Chem Soc 97:6866, 1975.
5. Hinshaw WS: Image formation by nuclear magnetic resonance: The sensitive point method. J Appl Phys 47:3709, 1976.
6. Damadian R, Minkoff L, Goldsmith M, et al: Tumor imaging in a live animal by field focusing NMR (FONAR). Physiol Chem Phys 8:61, 1976.
7. Damadian R: Tumor detection by nuclear magnetic resonance. Science 1977:1151, 1971.
8. Frey HE, Knispel RR, Kruuv J: Proton spin-lattice relaxation studies of nonmalignant tissues of tumorous mice. JNCI 49:903, 1972.
9. Inch WR, McCredie JA, Knispel RR, et al: Water content and proton spin relaxation time for neoplastic and non-neoplastic tissues from mice and humans. JNCI 52:353, 1974.
10. Coles BA: Dual-frequency proton spin relaxation measurements on tissues from normal and tumor-bearing mice. JNCI 57:389, 1976.
11. Edrich J, Hardee PC: Thermography at millimeter wavelengths. Proc IEEE 62:1391, 1974.

12. Edrich J: Microwave absorption of living human skin between 8 and 96 GHz. Proc 5th Europ Microwave Conf, Microwave Exhibitions and Publications LTD, England, September, 1975, pp 361–364.
13. Edrich J: Thermographic imaging at millimeter and centimeter wavelengths, in Gray J, Hendee WR (eds): Application of Optical Instrumentation in Medicine, IV. Palos Verdes Estates, Cal, Society of Photo-Optical Instrumentation Engineers, 1976.
14. Guy WA: Analyses of electromagnetic fields induced in biological tissues by thermographic studies on equivalent phantom models. IEEE Trans Microwave Theory Techniques MTT-19:205, 1971.
15. Barrett AH, Myers PC: Microwave thermography. Bibl Radiol 6:45, 1975.
16. Cacak RK, Winans DE, Edrich J, Hendee WR: Millimeter wavelength thermographic scanner. Med Phys, 8:462, 1981.
17. Carson PL, Oughton TV, Hendee WR, et al: Imaging soft tissue through bone with ultrasound transmission tomography by reconstruction. Med Phys 4:302, 1977.
18. Greenleaf JF, Johnson SA, Bahn RC, Rajogopalan B: Quantitative cross-sectional imaging of ultrasound parameters. 1977 Ultrasonics Symposium Proceedings, IEEE CAT 77CH1264–1SU, 1978.
19. Glover GH: Computerized time-of-flight ultrasonic tomography for breast examination. Ultrasound Med Biol 3:117, 1977.
20. Glover GH, Sharp JC: Reconstruction of ultrasound propagation speed distributions in soft tissue: Time-of-flight tomography. IEEE Trans Sonics Ultrasonics 24:229, 1977.
21. Greenleaf JF, Johnson SA, Samayoa WF, Duck FA: Algebraic reconstruction of spatial distributions of acoustic velocities in tissue from their time-of-flight profiles, in Booth H (ed): Acoustical Holography, vol 6. New York, Plenum Press, 1974, pp 71–90.
22. Hoop B, Burnham CA, Correll JE, et al: Myocardial imaging with $^{13}NH_4$ and a multicrystal positron camera. J Nucl Med 14:181, 1973.
23. Pentlow KS, Beattie JW, Laughlin JS: Parameters and design considerations for tomographic transmission scanners, in Ter-Pogossian MM, Phelps ME, Brownell GL, et al (eds): Reconstruction Tomography in Diagnostic Radiology and Nuclear Medicine. Baltimore, University Park Press, 1977, pp 267–279.
24. Brownell GL, Burnham CA, Chesler DA, et al: Transverse section imaging of radionuclide distributions in heart, lung, and brain, in Ter-Pogossian MM, Phelps ME, Brownell GL, et al (eds): Reconstruction Tomography in Diagnostic Radiology and Nuclear Medicine. Baltimore, University Park Press, 1977, pp 293–307.
25. Phelps ME, Hoffman EJ, Mullani NA, et al: Some performance and design characteristics of PETT III, in Ter-Pogossian MM, Phelps ME, Brownell GL, et al (eds): Reconstruction Tomography in Diagnostic Radiology and Nuclear Medicine. Baltimore, University Park Press, 1977, pp 371–392.
26. Cho ZH, Eriksson L, Chan J: A circular ring transverse axial positron camera, in Ter-Pogossian MM, Phelps ME, Brownell GL, et al (eds): Reconstruction Tomography in Diagnostic Radiology and Nuclear Medicine. Baltimore, University Park Press, 1977, pp 393–421.

TWO

X-Ray Transmission Computed Tomography

William R. Hendee

The detection and diagnosis of cancer by radiologic imaging techniques have improved significantly over the past few years, as conventional imaging procedures have improved in specificity and sensitivity and as new imaging technologies have entered the medical arena. For detection and diagnosis of any specific disease process, alternate pathways through the hierarchy of imaging techniques have been proposed from time to time. Usually, the choice of a particular pathway reflects the personal preference and bias of an individual physician rather than a well-conceived plan of attack based on an objective appraisal of the diagnostic yield of each step in the hierarchy of imaging methodologies. This approach not only is time-consuming and an inefficient use of medical equipment and personnel, it is also expensive and occasionally hazardous for the patient. In addition, this process makes the selection of imaging modalities vulnerable to rigid controls imposed by governmental regulatory agencies.

Because of the innovative character of x-ray transmission computed tomographic images and the necessity to justify the capitalization of equipment used to produce these images, computed tomography is particularly susceptible to patient application when other, less costly imaging techniques might be more appropriate. To identify the proper position of computed tomography within the hierarchy of imaging modalities in the detection and diagnosis of cancer, considerable effort is required. This effort must encompass a number of considerations, including the diagnostic information provided by computed tomography compared to that provided by alternate imaging modalities,[1-8] the sequence of imaging procedures which yields the most direct route to detection and diagnosis of pathology, and the cost and patient hazard of computed tomography compared to that of other imaging modalities.[9-12]

As part of this research effort, attention should be focused upon utilization of quantitative patient data provided by computed tomography as well as on the diagnostic efficacy of computed tomography relative to alternate imaging procedures for specific disease entities. To accomplish these objectives, research resources should be directed towards a number of projects as they pertain to computed tomography and its usefulness in cancer detection and diagnosis.

HISTORY AND CURRENT STATUS OF COMPUTED TOMOGRAPHY

Computed tomography entered the arena of radiologic imaging in the 1970s with an abruptness which is perhaps unparalleled in the history of medical imaging. Since its commercial introduction in 1972, computed tomography has evolved through four generations to its present status whereby high quality images are available in as short a time as 2 seconds. In all likelihood, the introduction of computed tomography will someday be heralded in radiology as the beginning of the era of computer data processing and soft copy formatting of images.

The process of image reconstruction from projections dates back to the early part of this century, when the mathematical fundamentals were described by the Austrian mathematician, Radon.[13] In the 1950s, image reconstruction techniques were applied in the fields of solar astronomy[14,15] and electron micrography.[16-18] The applicability of the technique to medical imaging remained essentially unrecognized, however, even though it was suggested by Oldendorf, a neurologist who constructed the first prototype transmission CT scanner in 1961.[19] Oldendorf's small-scale scanner consisted of a radioactive source and a scintillation detector with the object rotated between source and detector.

In the early 1960s, considerable effort was applied by Kuhl and Edwards to adapt the technique to image reconstruction from projections to problems in nuclear medicine.[20] These investigators initially used a simple back-projection approach of image reconstruction. The resulting blurring associated with this technique provided a fundamental handicap to its application to transmission imaging. On the other hand, Kuhl and Edwards are recognized as the undisputed originators of emission computed tomography.

In the late 1950s, Cormack, a physicist at the University of Capetown, became interested in the determination of attenuation coefficients across

cross-sectional planes of patients scheduled for radiation therapy. Cormack realized that a cross-sectional matrix of coefficients could be determined if measurements of x-ray transmission were obtained at many projections and angles through the body. He also realized that these coefficients could be displayed as a gray-scale visualization of internal anatomy. The first experimental verification of this approach utilized a collimated 7 mCi cobalt-60 (Co-60) source and a G-M counter as the detector. In 1957, Cormack moved to Tufts University in the United States, where he continued his work on image reconstruction, finally publishing two articles in the *Journal of Applied Physics*.[21,22] Unfortunately, these articles did not receive the attention they deserved.

Ten years after Cormack's initial studies, Hounsfield became interested in pattern recognition studies at the Central Research Laboratories of Electro-Musical Instruments Ltd. (EMI) in England. Like Cormack, Hounsfield speculated that the internal structure of the body could be reconstructed from a number of x-ray transmission measurements obtained tomographically.[23] He also calculated the theoretical accuracy of the technique and concluded that at acceptable dose levels it would be possible to measure the absolute value of x-ray attenuation coefficients with an accuracy of 0.5 percent.

Hounsfield's first apparatus was similar to Cormack's, except that an americium-241 (Am-241) source and a sodium iodide (NaI) detector were employed. Shortly thereafter, an x-ray tube was employed in place of the Am-241 source so that data could be obtained more rapidly. With this apparatus and the help of two radiologists, J. Ambrose and L. Kreel, images were obtained of a variety of biologic specimens.

The first computed tomographic scanner for clinical head scanning was installed in 1971 at the Atkinson Morley's Hospital in Wimbledon. The scanner employed synchronous translation of the x-ray source and NaI detector, with each translation occurring in a separate angular increment of 1° over a 180° arc. A water bag was positioned around the patient's skull to normalize the skull diameter in all directions. A total of 28,800 transmission measurements was obtained over a period of 4½ minutes, followed by another 20 minutes for image reconstruction. In April, 1972, clinical CT data were presented at the annual meeting of the British Institute of Radiology, followed by presentation of similar data that fall at the International Congress of Radiology and the Radiological Society of North America. Clinical data were first published in 1973.[24] Early in the summer of 1973, the first EMI head scanners arrived in North America for delivery to Massachusetts General Hospital, the Mayo Clinic, and the Montreal Neurological Institute.

As the EMI head scanner was being introduced in the clinical arena, R. Ledley of Georgetown University was developing the ACTA CT scanner for whole body as well as head examinations. This unit did not employ a water bath. The first commercial model of the ACTA scanner was installed in 1973 at the University of Minnesota.[25]

At the Cleveland Clinic in 1974, the prototype of the Ohio Nuclear CT Delta Scanner was evaluated clinically by Alfidi and associates.[26] Very quickly, many other companies, including all major manufacturers of x-ray equipment, initiated developmental programs in computed tomography, so that by 1976, 20 or so companies offered one or more models of computed tomographic equipment to the commercial marketplace. By 1980, this number of companies had decreased significantly as the financial strain of competing with major equipment manufacturers had been realized by smaller companies.

The first CT units employed a pencil beam of x-rays and a combination of translational and rotational motion for the x-ray tube and detector, as illustrated in Figure 2-1. These units are referred to as first generation CT scanners. Although first generation scanners provided excellent images of such structures as the head, where patient motion could be controlled, data collection times were measured in minutes and were unsatisfactory

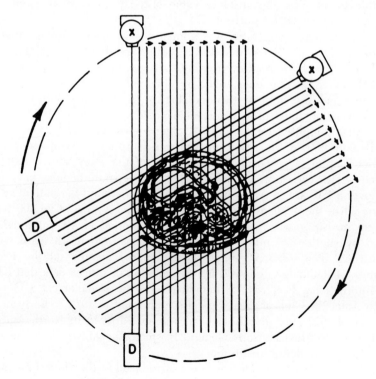

FIGURE 2-1. First generation CT scanner.

for anatomic regions where patient motion was significant. The first improvement in scanning geometry was achieved when a fan beam was substituted for the pencil beam of x-rays, as illustrated in Figure 2-2. This innovation was introduced in 1973 with the advent of the Ohio Nuclear Delta Scanner. Scanners utilizing this improvement in beam geometry are referred to as second generation CT scanners. With this feature, scan times were reduced from minutes to 20 seconds or so. Further reductions in scan time necessitated elimination of the translational motion of source and detector so that only rotation was employed in the acquisition of transmission data. The first purely rotational CT scanner was introduced by General Electric in 1975 (Fig. 2-3). This approach to CT imaging reduced scan times to as short as 2 seconds, and such devices are referred to as the third generation of CT scanners. In the General Electric scanner, a bank of ionization chambers is used as the detecting system in place of the scintillation detectors used in most computed tomographic units.

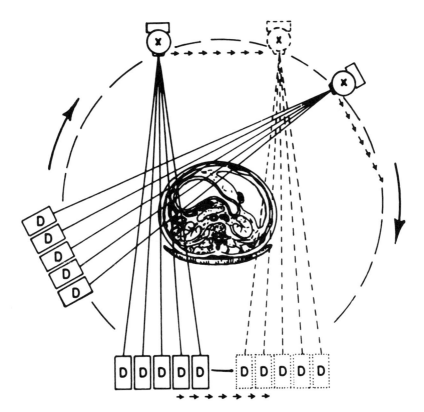

FIGURE 2-2. Second generation CT Scanner.

With financial assistance from the National Institutes of Health, an alternate approach to the design of a purely rotational CT scanner was revealed in 1976 by the American Science and Engineering Company of Cambridge, Massachusetts. This approach utilized a stationary array of 620 scintillation detectors surrounding the aperture where the patient is positioned. The x-ray tube rotates through 360° within the array, as illustrated in Figure 2-4. This approach also permits acquisition of all the projection data needed for an image in 2 seconds and allows normalization of the response of all detectors twice during each scan. The stationary array approach to CT imaging is termed a fourth generation design, although probably there are few, if any, clinical advantages of the fourth generation design over the third generation.

Although the evaluation of CT scanner design has proceeded at a remarkable pace over the past 8 years, the easy mechanical improvements have now been achieved and further innovations are likely to occur at a considerably slower rate. These innovations probably will be more in the software arena than in the hardware aspects of CT units and will be

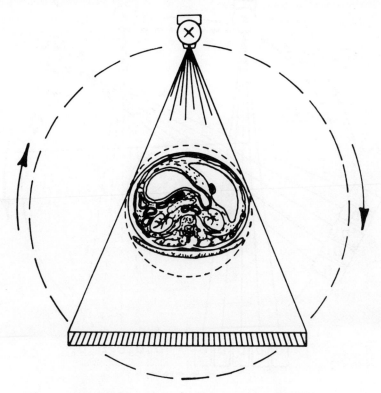

FIGURE 2-3. Third generation CT Scanner.

oriented primarily to reduction of image artifacts, improvements in low
contrast perceptibility, presentation of tomographic data in new formats,
and utilization of gating techniques to correlate data acquisition to physiologic variables. Software innovations already introduced with some scanners include the gray-scale visualization of longitudinal and oblique
sections, the display of quantitative tomographic data in histogram and
graphical formats, and the presentation of first- and higher-order differen-
tials of x-ray attenuation coefficients with respect to space and time
coordinates.

RECOMMENDATIONS FOR RESEARCH SUPPORT

*Physical Studies of Computed Tomography Compared to Alternate Imag-
ing Modalities.* This study would involve primarily phantom studies of
the ability to alternate imaging modalities to delineate pathologic conditions simulating those present in the cancer patient. Physical characteristics to be evaluated include low contrast perceptibility, the visibility of
anatomic detail, and the interference of structure and photon noise with

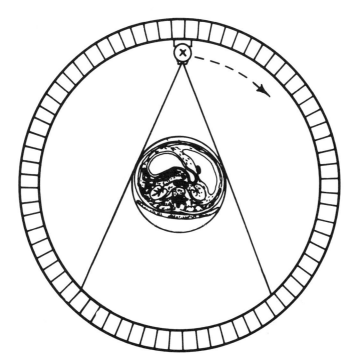

FIGURE 2-4. Fourth generation CT Scanner.

the visualization of patient pathology. The relationship of these characteristics to the visualization of patient pathology in clinical images should be delineated as an integral part of these studies. At present, the correlation between phantom studies and clinically significant information is obscure in most evaluations of radiologic imaging systems.

Priority: 1
Duration: 3 years
Probability of Success: excellent

Tissue Characterization Studies.   By utilizing quantitative data about patient composition which accompany gray-scale tomographic images, the characterization of tissue composition should be possible. This characterization should be exceptionally helpful in distinguishing normal from cancerous tissue. Aiding in this differentiation might be more sophisticated tissue characterization techniques, such as frequency spectrum analysis of transmitted x-rays, attenuation coefficient dispersion in regions of abnormal tissues, and multidimensional gradient analysis of coefficients across the patient cross-section. Before these techniques can be evaluated, certain inconsistencies in computed tomographic data must be resolved. Among these inconsistencies are x-ray beam hardening,[27,28] algorithm overshoot in regions of high density gradients,[29,30] photon noise and its contribution to imprecision of attenuation coefficients,[31-34] and frequency filtering of computed tomography reconstruction programs.

Priority: 1
Duration: 5 years
Probability of Success: moderate

Multicenter Efficacy Studies of Alternate Imaging Modalities.   To compensate for varying levels of computed tomographic capability among institutions and for the innate bias of individuals, multicenter studies are essential to identify the efficacy of computed tomography in comparison to alternate imaging modalities for particular disease processes. These studies must be designed with rigid protocols for patient admission and evaluation, and they must be conducted within the constraints of accepted statistical methods. Included in the multicenter studies should be an evaluation of the cost and patient risk of computed tomography in comparison to similar characteristics for other imaging modalities. Such an evaluation is exceptionally difficult, because it implies a quantitative appraisal of diagnostic information and yield time in relation to patient risk and the cost of diagnostic procedures. The difficulty of this evaluation is matched only by its need, and for that reason resources should be allocated to its pursuit. The need for these studies is acute, and they are in immediate need for funding.

Priority: 1
Duration: 5 years
Probability of Success: poor to good, depending on the
disease process

Use of Computed Tomography in Evaluating Response to Therapy. The potential of computed tomography as a mechanism with which to evaluate the progress of various therapeutic regimens is excellent. Considerable effort is already under way to assess this application of computed tomography in following the progress of patients over a course of radiation therapy, as well as in the comparative evaluation of alternate treatment plans for radiation therapy patients.[16,35-42] Stimulation of this effort by increased allocation of financial and manpower resources is recommended.

Priority: 2
Duration: ongoing
Probability of Success: moderate to excellent, depending on
the disease process and therapeutic regimen

Target Localization Techniques Utilizing Computed Tomography. The conjunction of computed tomography with stereotaxic immobilization techniques has the potential for improved target localization methods for stereotaxic surgery. This approach has been investigated in nonclinical surgical trials in combination with two- and three-dimensional computer graphics[43,44] and should be pursued at both investigational and clinical levels (Table 2-1).

Priority: 2
Duration: 3 to 5 years
Probability of Success: moderate to good

TABLE 2-1. SUMMARY OF RESEARCH RECOMMENDATIONS FOR TUMOR IMAGING WITH COMPUTED TOMOGRAPHY

Project	Priority	Duration (yr)	Probability of Success
Physical studies of computed tomography compared to alternate imaging modalities	1	3	Excellent
Tissue characterization studies	1	5	Moderate
Multicenter efficacy studies of alternate imaging modalities	1	5	Poor–good, depending on disease process
Use of computed tomography in evaluating response to therapy	2	Ongoing	Moderate–excellent, depending on disease process and therapeutic regimen
Target localization techniques utilizing computed tomography	2	3–5	Moderate–good

ACKNOWLEDGMENTS

Gratitude is expressed for contributions by Drs. A. E. James, Jr. and Craig Coulam from the Department of Radiological Sciences at Vanderbilt, as well as to Dr. P. Ruben Koehler, Department of Radiology at the University of Utah College of Medicine, for reviewing the manuscript of this chapter.

REFERENCES

1. Biello DR, Levitt RG, Siegel BA, et al: Computed tomography and radionuclide imaging of the liver: A comparative evaluation. Radiology 127:159, 1978.
2. Buell U, Kazner E, Rath M, et al: Sensitivity of computed tomography and serial scintigraphy in cerebrovascular disease. Radiology 131:393, 1979.
3. Carter BL, Kahn PC, Wolpert SM, et al: Unusual pelvic masses: A comparison of computed tomographic scanning and ultrasonography. Radiology 121:383, 1976.
4. Korobkin M, Callen PW, Filly RA, et al: Comparison of computed tomography, ultrasonography, and gallium-67 scanning in the evaluation of suspected abdominal abscess. Radiology 129:89, 1978.

5. Kressel HY, Margulis AR, Gooding GW, et al: CT scanning and ultrasound in the evaluation of pancreatic pseudocysts: A preliminary comparison. Radiology 126:153, 1978.

6. Levine, E, Lee KR, Neff JR, et al: Comparison of computed tomography and other imaging modalities in the evaluation of musculoskeletal tumors. Radiology 131:431, 1979.

7. Robbins AH, Pugatch RD, Gerzof SG, et al: Observations on the medical efficacy of computed tomography of the chest and abdomen. Am J Roentgenol 131:15, 1978.

8. Carter BL, Morehead J, Wolpert SM, et al: Cross-sectional Anatomy: Computed Tomography and Ultrasound Correlation. New York, Appleton–Century–Crofts, 1977.

9. Policy Implications of the Computed Tomography (CT) Scanner, Congress of the United States, Office of Technology Assessment, August 1978.

10. Evens RG, Jost RG: Utilization of head computed tomography units. Radiology 131:691, 1979.

10A. Evens RG, Jost RG: Utilization of body computed tomography units. Radiology 131:695, 1979.

11. Computed Tomographic Scanning, National Academy of Sciences Policy Statement, April 1977.

12. Wittenberg J, Fineberg HV, Black EB, et al: Clinical efficacy of computed body tomography. Am J Roentgenol 131:5, 1978.

13. Radon J: Ueber die Bestimmung von Funktionen durch ihre integralwerte laengs gewisser Mannigfaltigkeiten. (On the determination of functions from their integrals along certain manifolds.) Berichte Saechsische Adadamie der Wissenschaften (Leipzig) Mathematische–Physische Klasse 69:262, 1917.

14. Bracewell RN: Two-dimensional aerial smoothing in radio astronomy. Aust J Phys 9:297, 1956.

15. Branson NJBA: The emission spectrum of the Crab Nebula. Observatory 85:250, 1965.

16. Emami B, Melo A, Carter BL, et al: Value of computed tomography in radiotherapy of lung cancer. Am J Roentgenol 131:63, 1978.

17. Gilbert PFC: The reconstruction of a three-dimensional structure from projections and its application to electron microscopy: II. Direct methods. Proc R Soc Lond [Biol] 182:89, 1972.

18. Crowther RA, Amos LA, Finch JT, et al: Three dimensional reconstructions of spherical viruses by Fourier synthesis from electron micrographs. Nature 226:421, 1970.

19. Oldendorf W: Isolated flying spot detection of radiodensity discontinuities: Displaying the internal structural pattern of a complex object. IRE Trans Biomed Elec BME-8:68, 1961.

20. Kuhl DE, Edwards RQ: Image separation radioisotope scanning. Radiology 80:653, 1963.

21. Cormack AM: Representation of a function by its line integrals, with some radiological applications. J Appl Phys 34:2722, 1963.

22. Cormack AM: Representation of a function by its line integrals, with some radiological applications: II. J Appl Phys 35:2908, 1964.

23. Ambrose J: Computerized transverse axial scanning (tomography): Part 2. Clinical application. Br J Radiol 46:1023, 1973.

24. Hounsfield GN: Computerized transverse axial scanning (tomography): Part 1. Description of system. Br J Radiol 46:1016, 1973.

25. Ledley RS, DiChiro G, Luessenhop AJ, et al: Computerized transaxial x-ray tomography of the human body. Science 186:207, 1974.
26. Alfidi RJ, MacIntyre WJ, Meaney TF, et al: Experimental studies to determine application of CAT scanning to the human body. Am J Roentgenol 124:199, 1975.
27. Cacak RK, Hendee WR: Performance evaluation of a fourth generation computed tomography (CT) scanner. Proc SPIE 173:194, 1979.
28. Zatz LM, Alvarez RE: An inaccuracy in computed tomography: The energy dependence of CT values. Radiology 124:91, 1977.
29. Brooks RA, DiChiro G: Principles of computer assisted tomography (CAT) in radiographic and radioisotopic imaging. Phys Med Biol 21:689, 1976.
30. Glover GH, Eisner RL: Theoretical resolution of computed tomography systems. J Comput Assist Tomogr 3:85, 1979.
31. Brooks RA, DiChiro G: Statistical limitations in x-ray reconstructive tomography. Med Phys 3:237, 1976.
32. Chesler DA, Riederer SJ, Pelc NJ: Noise due to photon counting statistics in computed x-ray tomography. J Comput Assist Tomogr 1:64, 1977.
33. Huesman RH: The effects of a finite number of projection angles and finite lateral sampling of projections on the propagation of statistical errors in transverse section reconstruction. Phys Med Biol 22:511, 1977.
34. Wagner RF, Brown DG, Pastel MS: Application of information theory to the assessment of computed tomography. Med Phys 6:83, 1979.
35. Goitein M, Wittenberg J, Doucette J, et al: The value of CT in radiotherapy treatment planning. J Comput Assist Tomogr 2:524, 1978.
36. Goitein M: Computed tomography in planning radiation therapy. Int J Radiat Oncol Biol Phys 5:445, 1979.
37. Hendee WR: Computed tomography in radiation therapy treatment planning. Int J Radiat Oncol Biol Phys 4:539, 1978.
38. Hobday PA, Husband JE, Parker RP, et al: Radiotherapy treatment planning: Initial clinical experience using a whole body CT scanner directly linked to a treatment planning computer. J Comput Assist Tomogr 2:525, 1978.
39. Munzenrider JE, Pilepich M, Rene-Ferrero JB, et al: Use of body scanner in radiotherapy treatment planning. Cancer 40:170, 1977.
40. Ragan DP, Perez CA: Efficacy of CT-assisted two-dimensional treatment planning: Analysis of 45 patients. Am J Roentgenol 131:75, 1978.
41. Stewart JR, Hicks JA, Boone MLM, et al: Computed tomography in radiation therapy. Int J Radiat Oncol Biol Phys 4:313, 1978.
42. Yu WS, Sagerman RH, King GA, et al: The value of computed tomography in the management of bladder cancer. Int J Radiat Oncol Biol Phys 5:135, 1979.
43. Brown RA: A stereotactic head frame for use with CT body scanners. Invest Radiol 14:300, 1979.
44. Brown RA: A computerized tomography–computer graphics approach to stereotaxic localization. J Neurosurg 50:715, 1979.

THREE

Ultrasound

Marc S. Lapayowker, Marvin C. Ziskin, and Richard A. Banjavic

In a society concerned with integrating advanced scientific technology into the provision of better health care and more accurate medical diagnoses, the growth of diagnostic ultrasonic imaging has been a natural development. The use of ultrasound for diagnostic medical purposes has been under development since the late 1940s. Its medical use was an outgrowth of the development of metal flaw detectors and naval sonar during World War II and is attributed primarily to Drs. George Ludwig, Douglas Howry, and John Wild. The design of ultrasonic scanning equipment progressed rapidly from the B-29 gun turret model shown in Figure 3-1A and B constructed in 1951 by Howry.[1]

In this chapter, the present state of ultrasound as a diagnostic oncologic imaging modality is addressed together with recommendations for certain areas for further research.

STATUS OF ONCOLOGIC IMAGING

Physical Principles
Most ultrasound imaging techniques commonly used today for oncologic studies are based upon pulse-echo techniques. In this application, a directed, short-duration (about 2 or 3 cycles) pulse in the 1 MHz to 10 MHz range is directed into the patient. The device employed for this directional process is the ultrasonic transducer. Ultrasonic "echoes" originate by reflection and scatterings at discontinuities in acoustic impedances within the patient. These echoes are received by the same transducer and

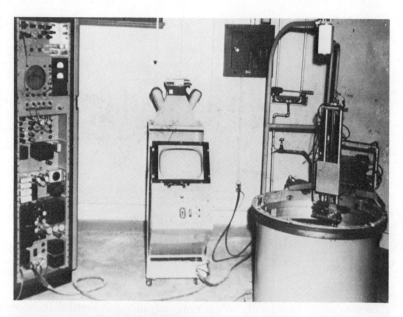

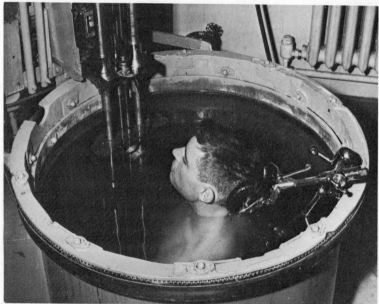

FIGURE 3-1. A: A B-29 gun turret scanner with electronic equipment is shown on the left, a display unit is shown in the center, and a scanning tank with rotating transducer mount is shown on the right. **B:** Patient immersed in gun turret for a scan of his neck. A lead weight is attached to the abdomen to prevent the patient from floating upwards.

are processed for display by subsequent electronic circuits. Because of geometric constraints, only those returning signals which are intercepted by the transducer are processed and displayed. In modern ultrasonic pulse-echo systems, the display unit provides either 16 or 32 levels of gray. The display level for a received echo, for a fixed position of the transducer, depends on the ratio of energy returned in the echo to the energy transmitted in the pulse. This ratio is critically dependent upon the fractional difference of the product of the physical mass density and acoustic speed of sound occurring at the discontinuity creating the returning signal. Figure 3-2 summarizes the nature of discontinuities common to medical scanning.

If the physical size of this discontinuity is larger than the interrogating beam diameter, as in Figure 3-2A, then the beam is reflected essentially in a specular fashion (i. e., the angle of reflection equals the angle of incidence). Boundaries of major organs or large neoplastic masses are examples of sources for specularly reflected echoes. In general, the relative strength of echoes reflected from these interfaces is large and frequency-independent, since the energy from the whole propagating beam is intercepted. The magnitude of the reflected echo depends on the angle of incidence of the ultrasound beam upon such an interface, with a maximum echo occurring when the beam impinges normally upon the interface. Work by some researchers has shown that for an inclination of 10° from the normal, a decrease of about 7 dB in scattered intensity amplitude is typical for biologically relevant interfaces.[2,3] This implies the obvious need for careful scanning techniques if the magnitude of specularly reflected echoes is to be used as a source of diagnostic information.

When the discontinuity is physically small compared to either the wavelength or the cross-section of the interrogating beam, one of several possible situations may result. If the discontinuity is a continuous interface, as in Figure 3-2B, diffuse reflection will occur. At normal incidence, echoes from diffuse reflection are smaller than specular reflections, since the energy is returned in a random fashion through all angles between 0° and ±90°. Echoes from these interfaces do not exhibit the strong angular dependence of specular reflections but may show a definite dependence on the frequency of the incident beam. In the case of Figure 3-2C, the discontinuities are not in the form of a continuous interface but rather appear as distinct entities. In this case, there is an extremely strong dependence of reflected echoes on the distribution of frequencies incident on the discontinuities. Since the frequency and wavelength are tied together by the speed of sound in the medium, there is also a dependence of the ultrasonic wavelength on the signal returned. In fact, it is the wavelength which becomes the "measuring stick" for the explanation of the relative size of the sources of scattering or their spatial arrangement.

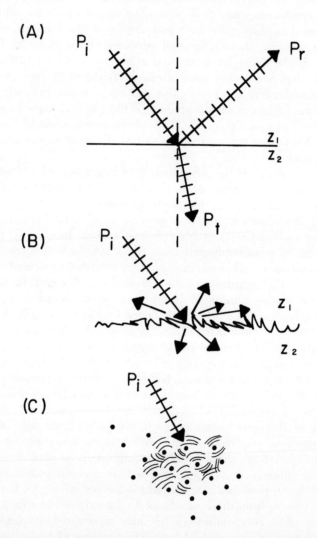

FIGURE 3-2. Possible arrangements of acoustic impedance discontinuities common in medical imaging. **A:** Large, smooth interface. **B:** Interface where the discontinuities are nonuniform and small with respect to the wavelength of the incident pulsed beam. **C:** A distribution of small discontinuities in a random, disjointed arrangement. For all three cases, P_i represents the incident pulsed beam, P_r the reflected pulsed beam, and P_t the transmitted beam. Z_1 and Z_2 are the acoustic impedances characteristic of either sides of a boundary interface.

For this case, then, the magnitude along with frequency distribution of the processed signals can provide diagnostic information.

In the case of moving discontinuities, the frequency spectrum of a reflected signal is shifted by the Doppler principle, whereby the amount of the shift is a function of the initial frequency of the beam, the speed of sound in the medium, and the relative velocity of the discontinuity with respect to the beam direction.[4] Most large interfaces in the body move at such slow speeds that the Doppler frequency shifts are less than a few hundred cycles per second and are difficult to detect. However, if the discontinuities causing the reflection are a collection of red blood cells moving through a vessel, then the Doppler shifts may be in the range of 0.8 to 8 kHz, depending on the flow conditions. Frequencies this high are within the range of human hearing and are easy to detect.

Available Instrumentation and Procedures
The current state of the art in diagnostic medical ultrasound is based primarily upon the use of the reflected ultrasound signals to furnish gray-scale images of internal structural interfaces and tissue parenchyma. The most common instrument is still the contact compound B-mode unit. The gray-scale images furnished by more recent B-mode units evidence a considerable advance over earlier black and white leading edge displays. Newer units have permitted the development of criteria for specific appearances of some organs and the evaluation of abnormalities seen within various organs and some neoplastic masses.[5,6] The advent in recent years of the digital scan converter as a replacement for the analog system has improved image quality and has resulted in even more characteristic appearances for various tissues and different disease states.[7] One of the main reasons for this improvement is that the electrical drift and over-write aspects of the analog systems are no longer problems with the digital scan converters. Most state of the art compound B-mode units in operation today employ a digital scan converter as part of their signal processing network. This feature has allowed extensive pre- and post-processing capabilities to be offered. These processing features permit the operator to expand or compress a chosen region of echo intensities over the gray-scale levels available in the display system.

B-mode image displays are only as good as the transducers which provide the acoustic information. Consequently, transducer technology has been expanding rapidly. There are now available a wide range of transducer probes using different center frequencies for broad-band pulses between 1.6 and 10 MHz. The use of focused transducers, including those focused both internally and externally, enables the sonographer to optimize the transducer chosen for the type of examination and the depth of the body part being examined.[8] Recently, the use of quarter-wavelength matching layers on the face of transducers has provided for more efficient sound transmission into the body.[9] This has allowed the use of higher frequency probes to maintain improved axial and lateral resolution without sacrificing sensitivity at depth. Compared to earlier transducers, the acoustic energy available now is not so severely limited by pulser excitation voltage or transducer inefficiency. An added development in contact compound imaging techniques is the availability of equal image quality real-time scanning instruments.[10,11] These instruments require an extremely short time for a complete scan, usually much less than a second. Scans are repeated at a very rapid rate and displayed continuously to form an image on a CRT or television monitor. Frame or image rates may vary from 15 to 150 scans per second without loss of resolution at the higher frame rates due to the interlacing of acoustic scan lines on the image.[12]

In real-time ultrasound scanning, there are four basic types of transducer operation: (1) mechanically rotating or sectoring, (2) multielement linear transducer arrays in which groups of elements are excited sequentially with a fixed time delay, (3) multielement arrays in which the timing of electronic excitation takes place in a multiplexed or phased fashion to allow beam steering or dynamic focusing, and (4) annular arrays. In the design of most of the mechanical arrays, a water-type standoff is used in the path between the transducer and skin surface so that probe motion does not cause undesirable movement artifacts from contact with the skin or body. Linear and phased arrays are in common usage today with many real-time systems, while annular arrays are employed only in one commercial scanner. Nevertheless, annular arrays are currently under extensive research and development.[13]

The current application of static and real-time instruments to oncologic imaging is widespread. Most of the present usage is devoted to evaluation of the retroperitoneal region, with emphasis on the imaging of abdominal organs for the presence and extent of tumors.[14,15] Ultrasound has been particularly valuable in differentiating between cystic and solid lesions.[16,17] Ultrasound also has been extremely valuable in a specific way regarding the presence and extent of lymphoma and metastatic disease,[18] the localization of tumors and follow-up of the results of their radiotherapeutic treatment,[19,20] visualization of the pancreas[21,22] and liver,[23,24] and particularly in evaluation of pelvic organs, masses, and fluid collections.[25,26] One area of investigation that should not be overlooked is the ability to investigate superficial lesions throughout the body. Oftentimes these lesions are roentgenographically invisible, so ultrasound has provided a singular means of imaging these masses.[27,28] A desirable application of real-time scanning is in the examination of the heart, where the presence or absence of abnormal masses can be appreciated when the heart is in motion.[29]

Some ultrasonic instrumentation is presently available which is specific to certain procedures. Doppler devices have been developed for observation and analysis of moving structures in the body, but just as important, there is the potential for the investigation of blood flow to and from a neoplastic mass as well as the acquisition of quantitative data describing vascular dynamics.[30,31] Newer high frequency transducers (above 9 MHz) are being employed to evaluate the presence of tumors in the retro-orbital area[32] and the posterior aspect of the globe of the eye,[33] where the acoustic window is ideal.

Another type of instrumentation has been moving out of the research phase and into assessment as a clinical tool. Through the use of a computer, a CT-type reconstruction algorithm allows the processing of data collected by through-transmission of acoustic pulses rather than reflection imaging.[34,35] A region of the body of particular practicability for this procedure is the breast, and the potential for identification and diagnosis of breast masses from ultrasonic through-transmission tomography is currently under active study.[36]

Limitations

A major problem relating to the use of ultrasound in general and in oncology in particular is the limited areas of the body which are accessible for imaging. Due to the nature of the acoustic interactions, regions containing or obscured by gas or air as well as regions in or obscured by bony structures are usually inaccessible. With the increased acoustic energy now available on clinical instruments, the ability to penetrate highly attenuating or reflective masses may exist; however, the lack of knowledge of the bioeffects of pulsed ultrasound at diagnostic intensity levels precludes this increase in transmitted power. The solution of technical problems related to acquiring better lateral and axial resolution on gray-scale images requires an increase in knowledge of the fundamental in vivo acoustic properties of tissues in order to understand what happens to a broad-band pulse as it propagates through tissue. Another area which has received very little attention up to now is the best manner of patient preparation for both providing the best possible acoustical windows for imaging and enhancing acoustic contrast by use of selected materials. Another area of question is the role of quantitative information in oncologic imaging. Presently, most diagnostic interpretations of echograms are dependent on the clinician's eye and memory recognition. A limitation to this decision process may be the absence of quantitative data regarding dynamic parameters of blood flow or categorization of so-called tissue signature records. Admittedly, in most cases the clinician is able to make a diagnosis from the qualitative image, but there are cases when further information could be very useful. For one thing, in oncologic imaging for the assessment of radiation therapy or chemotherapeutic regimens, there may be a large degree of information contained in the texture appearance of the echo signals returned from the neoplastic regions under treatment.[37,38]

RECOMMENDATIONS FOR RESEARCH SUPPORT

Bioeffects Research Pertaining to Pulsed Diagnostic Beam Intensity Levels. As the efficiency of sound transmission improves through transducer technology, more energy is available in the interrogating ultrasonic beams. However, the question of what is the threshold for biologic damage to the cells and tissues being sonified remains unanswered.[39] Techniques and equipment are now available to measure accurately the low intensity levels which are common to pulsed diagnostic beams.[40] Since clinical safety must remain an ongoing concern, especially for a modality which is claimed to be nondeleterious to the patient, more research efforts must be made into the bioeffects of pulsed as well as continuous wave beams at these levels. The search to localize a given marker or damage indicator for low level bioeffects is difficult, but necessary. Just as important is the need to provide reproducibility in studies, using any marker which is found. It is hoped that from such efforts a scientific basis can be formed for establishing ultrasonic exposure guidelines for both equipment manufacturers and governmental regulatory agencies. Since new equipment is being developed constantly, a long-term commitment must be given to this work.

Priority: 1
Duration: 5 years
Probability of Success: good

Establishment of a Basis for Tissue Signatures of Normal and Abnormal Tissues. At the present time, most diagnostic interpretation of oncologic images relies on recognition of nonuniformities, variation in echogenicity, or other changes in appearance or location of normal anatomic structures. Presently, samples of tissue must be taken from these areas to clearly differentiate the tissue from normal pathology by its morphologic characteristics, as observed microscopically. However, precise differentiation based on mechanical properties also appears possible. Because these mechanical properties can be determined by analyzing the manner in which an ultrasound beam is modified as it passes through tissue, they are commonly referred to as acoustic properties of the tissue. Acoustic properties include density, speed of sound, acoustic impedance, absorption, attenuation and its frequency dependence, and reflectivity, as determined by angular and back-scattering cross-sectional coefficients. This complex of values is thought to be unique for a tissue and thus is known as that tissue's acoustic signature.

Preliminary studies have shown significant differences in acoustic signatures between certain normal and malignant tissues.[41,42] One of the problems in attempting to use these signatures as a noninvasive biopsy technique is the paucity of in vivo values for these acoustic parameters on normal tissue. Recent reports have primarily contained in vitro data.[43,44] Since these parameters are known to change with temperature, blood flow, morbidity, etc., measurement techniques should be developed to acquire in vivo values. Once the deviation of normal values is established, abnormal tissue can be identified more readily. This also should be an ongoing project area, as the applications of this signature analysis are numerous. For example, one area presently being studied is how these acoustic properties are related to the texture appearance of B-mode echograms.[45,46] As this work progresses, it may lead to developments into other areas where oncologic imaging with ultrasound is presently only minor. One of these areas is radiotherapy, where modalities such as x-ray computed tomography are used extensively for treatment planning, but where ultrasound information may be useful in following the tumor's response to therapy and monitoring the treated region during follow-up examinations.[47,48]

Priority: 1
Duration: 3 to 5 years
Probability of Success: excellent

Studies into Optimization of Patient Preparation for Clinical Scanning. This area is one that has not received much attention but may provide solutions to some of the major limitations in routine examinations. The possible availability of an agent or means of absorbing or otherwise preventing gas from collecting in bowels would allow a better visualization of abdominal studies. Any promising ideas should be supported strongly. The procedures presently implemented for inpatient preparation have been assumed to be the best, but this should not prevent further research in this area. It would require only a short-term commitment and would certainly be worthwhile to perform a composite study of procedures in different institutions.

As the versatility and resolution limits of available instrumentation improve, the need for the development and study of effective ultrasound contrast agents becomes important. A few ultrasonic contrast materials have already been used. Indocyanine green, rapidly injected saline, ether, water, urine, and methyl cellulose have been used in specific applications.[49,50] Where applicable, they have been very useful and readily accepted in clinical practice. The search for new contrast agents and/or applications of these and others available should be pursued with high priority, keeping in mind the concept that an ultrasound examination should still remain as nontraumatic as possible.

Priority: 1.5
Duration: 1 to 2 years
Probability of Success: fair

Improvements in Display Systems and Artifact Recognition. The interpretation of oncologic images can only be as good as the manner in which the information passing through the transducer is processed and displayed. Industrial technology has been progressing rapidly in signal processing and display systems related to aerospace research, television and communications, and recently into digital radiography.[51] The possible application of this technology to echographic viewing merits some investigation. For example, since the ultrasonic scanning procedure is indeed a three-dimensional process, the possible three-dimensional display of this information is worthy of investigation. This may be particularly useful for visualizing narrow, tortuous structures which are not confined to a single plane and thus are difficult to appreciate in serial views. To date, three-dimensional viewing systems have been rather awkward and have not generally been accepted. New ideas in this area should be given consideration.

In terms of two-dimensional systems, any developments which increase the dynamic range of the available gray-scale in the display or hard copy reproduction of that display should be investigated, since in most cases the display system is the limiting element of the ultrasonic instrument's signal-processing chain. Even with the optimization of the display system, the image must then be stored on film or video tape for clinical evaluation. All of today's hard copy devices can be improved significantly to give a better reproduction of the instrument's display system. A serious limitation existing in most real-time systems is the serious degradation of the image quality when other than video tape hard copies are employed. This should be studied in terms of both the instrument design and the hard copy devices used. Any improvements in the quality of the appearance of the echographic signals would show immediate rewards in providing a more scientific basis for otherwise qualitative echographic interpretation. This would occur by improving the relationship between the physical properties of tissue and their sonographic appearances on a B-scan, by better elucidation of the presence and origin of artifacts on B-scans,[46] and by allowing more precise physical measurements to be performed on echograms. This by its nature is a research area which does not show immediate promise of success but should be considered in any long-term support commitments.

Priority: 2
Duration: 5 to 7 years
Probability of Success: moderate

Exploration into Quantitative Imaging Procedures.   This section by its very nature is quite broad. In order to make any meaningful recommendation, only two areas will be specifically cited. The first regards the role of computers for enhancement of presently obtained diagnostic images and the second is the generation of oncologic images based upon a strictly numerical or digital format.

The first and foremost scientific instrument which is used in making diagnostic decisions based on ultrasonic oncologic images is the clinician's eye–brain network. The whole concept of quantitative imaging should be approached with this idea in mind. However, part of the advances in diagnostic ultrasound equipment available to the clinician has been the common appearance of digital scan converters, which in essence can be likened to minicomputers. With this device, both pre- and postprocessing abilities are now present. Some of this processing, such as beam and transducer compensation, appears to be on a rational basis and obviously worthwhile. Other forms of processing, particularly postprocessing, are of an *ad hoc* nature and need to be evaluated for their diagnostic efficacy. Because this processing directly modifies the sonographic image upon which the diagnostic interpretation is made, there must be a rationale established for its use. However, there may well be a case of diminishing returns for research support in this area, as has been experienced for image processing in other oncologic imaging modalities. The role of the computer in CT imaging, for example, should not necessarily be used as a blank check for the equivalent use of computers in the ultrasound image development chain. The quantification of echo patterns from within organs and tissues should be studied in light of the additional information it may provide the clinician in his/her decision-making process. Even though estimates of reflectivity and attenuation may be determined for selected regions of view on an echogram, much of the work still needs to be done to determine the meaningfulness and the usefulness of these numerical data.

One area which should be explored is the possibility of using image subtraction techniques in ultrasound similar to those used in digital fluoroscopy.[51] Perhaps through the use of different frequency images or different gain on images, subtraction may lead to improvements in the complications caused by bowel gas or bone blocking the acoustic windows, elimination of reverberations or other multiple reflection artifacts, or emphasis of acoustic enhancement or shadowing effects, which are often very important in clinical diagnoses.[45] Some success for this determination will likely occur within 2 to 4 years.

There is also a need to continue to study computer techniques which provide an alternative form of image display to standard pulse-echo views. One area that is showing itself worthy of support is through-transmission imaging.[34-36] Although it is somewhat limited in terms of the body regions accessible for imaging, the preliminary results in studies of neoplastic regions of the breast indicate characteristic values for speeds of sound and attenuation coefficients.[52] The continuation· of this work is necessary, especially in light of information on the increased incidence of cancer associated with mammographic studies in women under 40 years of age. At all times, however, any quantitative imaging scheme employing computers should be judged on the basis of the additional information it can provide to the clinician relative to what is available via more direct means or other oncologic imaging modalities.

Priority: 1
Duration: 2 to 4 years
Probability of Success: very good

Transducer Technology. The ultrasonic transducer is one of the most important components in ultrasonic instrumentation for obtaining echo information. Furthermore, many, if not most, instrumentation advances are in fact advances in transducer design. This is an ongoing endeavor and should be supported to encourage new developments in the foreseeable future. Industry, of course, can be expected to be a major contributor. Nevertheless, because of the transducer's importance to any advances in oncologic imaging and since developments in noncommercial research laboratories may provide the breeding ground for generation of fundamental concepts and feasibility studies, this work should receive the highest priority at all levels. One example of this noncommercial impetus was in the development of a real-time transducer for ultrasonically guided aspiration biopsy of neoplastic lesions.[53] The whole area of real-time scanning generates the need for development of improved multielement, multidimensional arrays for dynamic focusing capabilities both in and out of the main scan plane. The investigation of the ability of imaging by performing multifrequency transmission and reflection pulsing from a single transducer or several closely matched transducers may be an interesting project, since little attention has been paid to this concept in diagnostic instruments. Varying frequency narrow-band echo networks provide exquisitely sensitive target discrimination for such animals as bats and dolphins. Transducers capable of producing varying frequency signals may be useful for similar discrimination in oncologic imaging procedures and deserve investigation. Some consideration should also be given to projects incorporating transducers which are capable of *both* Doppler recording of flow or motion *and* B-mode imaging.[31] Commercial instruments are now available which are designed for both carotid and other peripheral vascular cross-sectional imaging. Soon to be released are devices which also have the capability of providing quantitative information about flow conditions and characteristics by using either the same imaging transducers or additional transducers for pulsed Doppler directional measurements. The cross-sectional images will allow the exact location of the source of the Doppler signals to be easily selectable. This may provide a means of evaluation of superficial tumors and their vascularization.[31] Any possible applications to oncologic imaging employing these devices should be given a high priority.

Priority: 1
Duration: 1 to 5 years
Probability of Success: excellent

ACKNOWLEDGMENTS

The authors wish to thank and acknowledge the following individuals for their contribution to the development of the ideas and preparation of this manuscript:

- Bruce D. Doust, M.D.
- Barry Goldberg, M.D.
- Raymond Gramiak, M.D.
- William R. Hendee, Ph.D.

• Donald L. King, M.D.
• Edward A. Lyons, M.D.
• Carol M. Rumack, M.D.
• Renate L. Soulen, M.D.
• William B. Steel, M.D.

REFERENCES

1. Holmes JH: Diagnostic ultrasound during the early years of A.I.U.M. JCU 8:299, 1980.
2. Kossoff G: Display techniques in ultrasound pulse echo investigations: A review. JCU 2:61, 1974.
3. Braun M, Robinson DE: Model studies of angular behavior of acoustic back-scatter. Ultrasound Med Biol 6:377, 1980.
4. Wells PNT: Ultrasonic Biophysics. New York, Academic Press, 1977.
5. Kossoff G, Garrett WJ, Carpenter DA, et al: Principles and classification of soft tissues by grey scale echography. Ultrasound Med Biol 2:89, 1976.
6. Taylor KJW, Carpenter DA, Hill CR, et al: Gray scale ultrasound imaging: The anatomy and pathology of the liver. Radiology 119:415, 1976.
7. Susal AL, Walker JT, Meindl JD: Small-organ dynamic imaging system. JCU 8:421, 1980.
8. Reid MH: Improved ultrasound image detail using wide aperture, focused transducers. Radiology 136:473, 1980.
9. Schuette WH, Shawker TH, Hall TE: Evaluation of a quarter wavelength matching layer transducer in abdominal scanning. JCU 7:65, 1979.
10. Maginness MG, Plummer JD, Beaver WL, Meindl JD: State-of-the-art in two-dimensional ultrasonic transducer array technology. Med Phys 3:312, 1976.
11. Macovski A: Ultrasonic imaging using arrays. Proc IEEE 67:484, 1979.
12. Meindl JD, Macovski A: Recent advances in the development of new imaging techniques, in White DN (ed): Recent Advances in Ultrasound in Bio-medicine. Forest Grove, Ore, Research Studies Press, 1977, pp 175–201.
13. Volkomerson D, Hurley B: Progress in annular-array imaging, in Booth N (ed): Acoustical Holography. New York, Plenum Press, 1975, vol 6, pp 145–164.
14. Schabel SI, Rittenberg GM, Bubanj R, et al: Pedunculated gastric leiomyoma: A wandering abdominal mass demonstrated by ultrasound. JCU 7:211, 1979.
15. Behan M, Kazam E: Echographic characteristics of fatty tissues and tumors. Radiology 129:143, 1978.
16. Thurber LA, Cooperberg PL, Clement JG, et al: Echogenic fluid: A pitfall in the ultrasonographic diagnosis of cystic lesions. JCU 7:273, 1979.
17. Goldberg BB, Kotler MN, Ziskin MC, Waxham RD: Diagnostic Uses of Ultrasound. New York, Grune and Stratton, 1975.
18. Hillman BJ, Haber KH: Echographic characteristics of malignant lymph nodes. JCU 8:213, 1980.
19. Banjavic RA, Tolbert DD, Zagzebski JA: ULTRACOMP: A computerized-operating system for the effective use of sonographic contour information in radiotherapy treatment planning. J Appl Radiol 6:135, 1977.

20. Heimburger RF, Eggleton RC, Fry FJ: Ultrasonic visualization in determination of tumor growth rate. JAMA 224:497, 1973.
21. Arger PH, Mulhern CB, Bonavita JA, et al: An analysis of pancreatic sonography in suspected pancreatic disease. JCU 7:91, 1979.
22. Doust BD, Pearce JD: Gray-scale ultrasonic properties of the normal and inflamed pancreas. Radiology 120:653, 1976.
23. Taylor KJW, Sullivan D, Rosenfield AT, et al: Gray scale ultrasound and isotope scanning: Complementary techniques for imaging the liver. AJR 128:277, 1977.
24. Reid MH: Visualization of the bile ducts using focused ultrasound. Radiology 118:155, 1976.
25. Miskin M, Martin B, Bain J: Ultrasonographic examination of scrotal masses. J Urol 117:243, 1977.
26. Engel JM, Deitch EA· Omentum mimicking cyctic masses in the pelvis. JCU 8:31, 1980.
27. Mettler FA, Schultz K, Kelsey CA, et al: Gray scale ultrasonography in the evaluation of neoplastic invasion of the base of the tongue. Radiology 133:781, 1979.
28. Feinberg S: Use of imaging techniques in cancer diagnosis. Minn Med 62:489, 1979.
29. Hibi N, Fukui Y, Nishimura K, et al: Real time observation of left atrial myxoma with high speed B-mode echocardiography. JCU 7:34, 1979.
30. Jonkman EJ: Doppler research in the 19th century. Ultrasound Med Biol 6:1, 1980.
31. White DN, Cledgett PR: Breast carcinoma detection by ultrasonic Doppler signals. Ultrasound Med Biol 4:329, 1978.
32. Skalka HW, Callahan MA, Elsas FJ: Echographic appearance of recurrent orbital retinoblastoma. JCU 8:164, 1980.
33. Restori M, McLeod D, Wright JE: Diagnostic ultrasound in ophthalmology. J R Soc Med 73:273, 1980.
34. Dick DE, Carson PL, Bayly EJ, et al: Technical evaluation of an ultrasound CT scanner. 1977 Ultrasonics Symposium Proceedings, IEEE Cat. No. 77CH1264-1SU, 1978.
35. Wilson RL: Ultrasonic tomography. Medicamundi 22:48, 1977.
36. Weiss L, Rosner D, Glenn WE: Visualization of breast lesions with an advanced ultrasonic device: Results of a pilot study. J Surg Oncol 10:251, 1978.
37. Leeman S, Badcock PC, Gore JC, et al: Ultrasonic backscattering assessment of tumour response to treatment. RPMS Medical Physics Report US78/1, Hammersmith Hospital, London, 1978.
38. Plessner J, Badcock PC, Leeman S: The accuracy of ultrasound scanning for radiotherapy field planning. Paper presented at Tumour Ultrasound '77, London, 1977.
39. Veluchamy V: Medical ultrasound and its biological effects. J Clin Engineering 3:162, 1978.
40. Baboux JC, Lakestani F, Perdrix M: Measurement of the ultrasonic energy radiated by transducers used in echography. Ultrasound Med Biol 5:75, 1979.
41. Calderon C, Vilkomerson D, Mezrich R, et al: Differences in the attenuation of ultrasound by normal, benign, and malignant breast tissue. JCU 4:249, 1976.
42. Goss SA, Frizzell LA, Dunn F: Ultrasonic absorption and attenuation in mammalian tissues. Ultrasound Med Biol 5:181, 1979.

43. Goss SA, Johnston RL, Dunn F: Comprehensive compilation of empirical ultrasonic properties of mammalian tissues. J Acoust Soc Am 64:423, 1978.
44. Goss SA, Johnston RL, Dunn F: Compilation of empirical ultrasonic properties of mammalian tissues: II. J Acoust Soc Am 68:93, 1980.
45. Kobayashi T: Diagnostic ultrasound in breast cancer: Analysis of retrotumorous echo patterns correlated with sonic attenuation by cancerous connective tissue. JCU 7:471, 1979.
46. Jaffe CC, Harris BS: Physical factors influencing numerical echo-amplitude data extracted from B-scan ultrasound images. JCU 8:327, 1980.
47. Brascho DJ: Tumor localization and treatment planning with ultrasound. Cancer (suppl) 39:697, 1977.
48. Zagzebski JA, Wiley AL, Tolbert DD, et al: Ultrasonic B-scanning for radiation therapy planning and follow-up of superficial tumors. Int J Radiat Oncol Biol Phys 2:715, 1977.
49. Meltzer RS, Tickner EG, Sahines TP, et al: The source of ultrasound contrast effect. JCU 8:121, 1980.
50. Black EB, Ferrucci JT Jr, Wittenberg J, et al: Acoustic contrast enhancement: Value of several system gain variations in gray scale ultrasonography. AJR 133:689, 1979.
51. Kruger RA, Mistretta CA, Crummy AB, et al: Digital K-edge subtraction radiography. Radiology 125:243, 1977.
52. Duck FA, Hill CR: Mapping True Ultrasonic Backscatter and Attenuation Distributions in Tissue—A Digital Reconstruction Approach. Second NBS Ultrasonic Tissue Characterization Symposium, NBS Special Publication 525, 1979, pp 247–251.
53. Saitoh M, Watanabe H, Ohe H, et al: Ultrasonic real time guidance for percutaneous puncture. JCU 7:269, 1979.

FOUR

Nuclear Medicine

Paul B. Hoffer, Alexander Gottschalk,
Barry Siegel, Leonard Freeman,
William Strauss, and Christopher C. Kuni

Nuclear imaging is still a developing technology. Although nuclear imaging methods currently play an important role in the diagnosis and monitoring of treatment of cancer, current methods do not exploit the full potential of the technology. Major areas of investigation and potential progress include determining the efficacy of current imaging methods, developing new radiopharmaceuticals and better methods for imaging these as well as conventional agents, determining the changes induced in scan images by treatment, and determining the role of other adjunctive imaging procedures used in combination with nuclear imaging. The projects proposed in this section are directed primarily toward these areas.

STATE OF THE ART

Efficacy Studies
There is a definite need to study the efficacy of radionuclide procedures which are designed to detect, stage, and follow the progression of cancer. Some efficacy studies have been carried out successfully on an independent basis.[1,2] However, such studies are best conducted in association with broader, disease-oriented clinical investigations.[3] Unfortunately, many clinically disease-oriented projects sponsored by the National Cancer Institute have either neglected or improperly utilized radionuclide imaging methods. In some cases they have used techniques which do not represent the state of the art at the time of the study. As a result, an opportunity to collect valuable information regarding the efficacy of vari-

ous nuclear imaging methods has been lost. Furthermore, some of the information which has been gathered is potentially misleading.

Development of New Tumor-imaging Agents and Better Understanding of the Modes of Action of Existing Agents

In the past, the detection of tumors by radionuclide imaging has depended chiefly on an assessment of the effects of the tumor on normal tissue—e.g., technetium-99m sulfur colloid (Tc-99m sc) imaging for hepatic tumors and Tc-99m phosphate imaging for detection of reactive changes accompanying bone tumors—or on the accumulation of certain radiopharmaceuticals in tumor tissue, a characteristic which has often been recognized only serendipitously—e.g., gallium-67 citrate (Ga-67 citrate). These approaches suffer from an inherent limitation in specificity and have not proven to be completely satisfactory for clinical evaluation of patients with known or suspected tumors. There is a need to develop new tumor-imaging agents based on known physiologic and immunologic aspects of tumor tissue. Some initial progress using radiolabeled antibodies to tumor antigen has already been made.[4–10]

The mechanisms by which currently available tumor-imaging agents localize are incompletely understood. Further elucidation of these mechanisms may be helpful in improving the quality of images obtained with these agents and uncovering unsuspected metabolic pathways which may be critical to tumor growth. For example, prior studies have shown that Ga-67 is largely bound to plasma proteins and is associated with lysosomal fractions of tumor tissue homogenates.[11] More recent evidence suggests that Ga-67 binds with high affinity to lactoferrin[12] and has other similarities to ferric ion. Localization of Ga-67 in tumors may provide some insight into the importance of ferric ion accumulation in tumors. Other tumor-seeking agents include cobalt-57 (Co-57) bleomycin,[13] glucose analogs,[14] Tc-99m tetrasulfophthalocyanine,[15] and iodine-131 DNase (I-131 DNase).[16]

It is also important to develop new general methods of attaching radionuclides to specific molecules which may localize in tumor. Currently, tumor-imaging agents are limited to radioactive ions (e.g., Ga-67 and I-131) and to compounds which are easily labeled due to their affinity for metal ions (e.g., Co-57 bleomycin). If labeling methods for tagging key compounds with physically suitable radionuclides could be developed, many potentially useful compounds (e.g., adriamycin) could be explored for tumor imaging.

Instrumentation

Improved detection of radionuclides is as important as the development of new imaging agents. A major area of recent development in nuclear imaging is the concept of quantitative imaging made possible by emission computed tomography (ECT). The development of ECT imaging has been spurred by the success of transmission computed tomography (TCT). The two techniques are similar in regard to the mathematics of reconstruction. The combination of the two techniques may be particularly powerful.

Kuhl and Edwards first introduced the concept of emission computed tomography in 1963 with their Mark I brain scanner.[17] This unit was subsequently updated to the current Mark IV system described in 1976.[18] Anger, in the mid 1960s, devised a linear emission tomographic system which has become commercially available.[19] This device has shown definite clinical utility as the instrument of choice for Ga-67 imaging.[20] Recently, rapid progress has also been made in the development of positron emission tomographic devices. Progress in this area includes the developments of Brownell, TerPogossian, Kuhl, and Phelps, as well as others as described in the review of positron tomography by Phelps.[21]

ECT devices which are built to utilize positrons are significantly different from those devices designed to detect single photon events. Reconstruction using positron emitters is somewhat easier, since these isotopes emit annihilation radiations which travel in almost exactly opposite directions. Therefore, it is possible to reconstruct the line on which the event occurred. Furthermore, positron-emitting isotopes are the only radioactive forms of a number of important physiologic elements, including oxygen, nitrogen, and fluorine. The major disadvantage of the positron system is the fact that most positron-emitting radionuclides of physiologic significance have a short half-life. They must therefore be produced by an on-site cyclotron. Tomographic reconstruction using single photon-emitting radionuclides requires somewhat more sophisticated techniques which take attenuation factors into account. However, there is a greater variety of radioisotopes and radiopharmaceuticals available for such studies.

Further instrumentation development in both areas of emission computed tomography is highly desirable. For example, prototype instruments designed for tomographic reconstruction using positrons have proved extremely useful in the critical evaluation of brain physiology in various diseases.[21] Application of both positron-imaging techniques and single photon radionuclide emission tomography for evaluation of tumor physiology and detection of metastasis would be important in the better understanding and treatment of cancer. A second function of these techniques would be the detection and sizing of primary tumors. Furthermore, the methods would also be helpful in determining which portion of the tumor mass is physiologically active and which portion is necrotic. Instrumentation and methods of this sort would also be extremely useful in evaluating effects of chemotherapeutic agents and other forms of treatment, such as radiation.

Evaluation of the Effects of Treatment on Scan Images

While nuclear imaging methods are used to follow the progress of treatment of cancer, the effects of the treatment modalities on the scanning agents themselves is incompletely understood. For example, bone scanning is a highly sensitive method for the detection of bone metastasis. It is frequently used to study the response of cancer to therapy.[22] However, relatively little is known regarding the precise correlation of bone scan changes and healing in metastatic lesions. Since the bone scan measures the response of bone to the destructive process rather than the destructive process itself, increased radionuclide uptake following therapy could indicate either extension or healing of the disease process.

Utilization of Adjunctive Procedures

As various imaging modalities develop, there is a tendency to look at each independently rather than as part of a complete diagnostic armamentarium. However, there are several areas in nuclear imaging where combined utilization of imaging procedures is perhaps indicated but incompletely explored.

Solitary bone lesions detected by radionuclide imaging in patients with known cancer represent a diagnostic enigma. It has been shown that about one-half of such solitary lesions are due to benign disease.[23] However, it is not clear whether it is safe to assume, when a patient has such a solitary lesion and the bone radiography is normal, that the lesion is due to a malignant process. It would be helpful to confirm bone destruction in such areas by a second modality before assuming a metastatic etiology.

Currently, the radionuclide liver scan is the primary method of detection of metastasis to this organ. However, the limitations of this study in both sensitivity and specificity are well documented.[1] While great progress has been made in the development of gray-scale imaging in ultrasonography, the sensitivity of this method compared to that of radionuclide imaging for detection of hepatic lesions is still unknown. It is unclear whether ultrasonography should be used routinely in addition to radionuclide imaging for evaluation for all patients in the assessment of the liver for metastasis or whether the study should be restricted to selected patients in whom abnormalities or "suspicious areas" are detected on the radionuclide liver scan.[24]

The radionuclide thyroid scan has been the primary imaging procedure for the evaluation of palpable thyroid nodules. It is also used to detect occult thyroid cancer in individuals with a history of thyroid radiation. If a palpable thyroid nodule is isotopically "cold" using either radioiodine or $^{99m}TcO_4$ as the imaging agent, there is approximately a 20 percent probability of the nodule harboring a malignancy. The incidence of thyroid cancer in isotopically warm or hot nodules is considerably lower. To date, ultrasonography has been used primarily to determine if isotopically cold nodules are cystic (low probability of cancer) or solid (higher probability of cancer). Recent technologic advances in ultrasonography include the development of small-area high-resolution transducers. It is possible that these devices will be as sensitive as and more specific than radionuclide methods in detecting thyroid cancer. A comparable study using both imaging modalities is required in this area also. A recent report suggests that thallium may be useful in the diagnosis of thyroid cancer.[25]

RECOMMENDATIONS FOR RESEARCH SUPPORT

Implementation of Improved Efficacy Studies as Part of NCI Diagnostic Protocols. All clinical study proposals which involve nuclear diagnostic procedures for detection, staging, or clinical follow-up of malignant disease should be reviewed by either individuals or groups who are experts in nuclear medicine procedures related to the malignancy or organ system under investigation. One way of implementing this review process would be to appoint a Nuclear Medicine Advisory Committee to the National Cancer Institute for purposes of clinical trial reviews. The Advisory Committee could provide a list of expert nuclear medicine reviewers for specific clinical projects, monitor the quality of nuclear medicine efficacy data being obtained from clinical studies, and make general recommendations to the individual project directors.

Priority: 1
Duration: ongoing
Probability of Success: high

Tumor-imaging Agents: Development of New Tumor-seeking Radiolabeled Compounds. One approach toward improving imaging is the synthesis of radiopharmaceuticals with biochemical specificity. Agents in this class include radiolabeled antibodies directed against tumor antigens, hormone analogs or hormone receptor antagonists, and enzyme inhibitors. Potential areas worthy of study include the development of estrogen receptor antagonists to permit the in vivo determination of breast carcinoma estrogen dependency. Another fruitful avenue might be the development of an inhibitor of ornithine decarboxylase. This enzyme is the rate-limiting enzyme in the polyamine biosynthetic pathway involving sequential formation of putrescine, spermine, and spermidine. The polyamines are found in high concentrations in rapidly dividing cell lines, in most tumors, in some normal tissues (pancreas, prostate), and in areas of rapid protein synthesis. The radiolabeled antibody approach is quite appealing and has been preliminarily investigated by several groups.[4,5] Further investigation is required to achieve higher antibody specificity, perhaps using hybridoma systems, to develop more suitable protein labels with better characteristics for imaging and to determine whether there are antigens specific to classes of human tumors.[26]

Priority: 1
Duration: 4 to 6 years
Probability of Success moderate

Tumor-imaging Agents: Characterization of the Mechanism of Localization of Tumor-seeking Radionuclides.   Mechanisms by which currently useful tumor-scanning agents localize must be further explored. Specifically, Ga-67, indium-111 (In-111), and ytterbium-169 (Yb-169), as well as other rare earth elements, should be investigated.

Priority: 1
Duration: 3 to 4 years
Probability of Success: high

Tumor-imaging Agents: Indirect Labeling of Biologically Active Molecules.   Chelate-containing derivatives of biologically active molecules should be developed which will chelate radionuclides irrespective of the parent compound. Such derivatives must not interfere with those functional groups which interact with the active site. Thus a major problem will be to design chelation groups which do not interfere with the biologic activity of the parent molecule.

This approach has general applicability to labeling of proteins (antibodies, polypeptide hormones), chemotherapeutic agents, and many other classes of drugs and/or biologically active compounds.

Priority: 1
Duration: 3 to 5 years
Probability of Success: high

Instrumentation: Tomographic Imaging Devices.   Progress in and development of positron emission detecting systems are already substantial.

Prototype devices are actually in use. Further use of these devices in studying physiologic processes relating to cancer must be encouraged. Development of single photon emission detection devices (except those for the head) is still in its infancy. These devices should be developed to their full clinical potential.

Priority: 1
Duration: 5 years
Probability of Success: high

Effects of Treatment on Radionuclide Images: Bone Imaging.   Numerous clinical studies are now in progress to determine the effects of various therapeutic modalities on cancer with osseous spread. Appropriate bone imaging and quantitative uptake studies should be performed on these patients in order to determine the temporal correlation of radionuclide bone uptake with Tc-99m phosphate agents and the progress of bone metastasis.

Priority: 2
Duration: 3 years
Probability of Success: high

Utilization of Adjunctive Imaging Procedures: Ultrasound and Radionuclide Methods.   A broad clinical study should be instituted to evaluate patients with known primary tumors for hepatic metastasis using both nuclear imaging and ultrasound. The relative value of each modality should be determined for specific tumor types.

A second clinical study should be instituted to compare radionuclide thyroid imaging with high-resolution ultrasound thyroid imaging for specificity in identifying the etiology of thyroid nodules.

Priority: 2
Duration: 2 years
Probability of Success: high

Utilization of Adjunctive Imaging Procedures: Use of Conventional X-ray and Computed Tomography to Determine the Etiology of Solitary Bone Scan Abnormalities.   A study of solitary bone lesions in patients with tumor, using both conventional radiographic tomography imaging systems and computed tomography, is required. Computed tomography may be capable of confirming localized bone destruction in many cases in which conventional radiography would not be adequately sensitive.

Priority: 3
Duration: 2 years
Probability of Success: moderate

REFERENCES

1. Drum DE, Christacopoulos JS: Hepatic scintigraphy in clinical decision making. J Nucl Med 13:908, 1972.
2. McNeil BJ, Hessel SJ, Branch WT, et al: Measures of clinical efficacy: III. The value of the lung scan in the evaluation of young patients with pleuritic chest pain. J Nucl Med 17:163, 1976.
3. DiMagno EP, Malagelada JR, Taylor WF, et al: A prospective comparison of current diagnostic tests for pancreatic cancer. N Engl J Med 297:737, 1977.
4. Hoffer PB, Lathrop K, Bekerman C, et al: Use of ^{131}I-CEA antibody as a tumor scanning agent. J Nucl Med 15:323, 1973.
5. Goldenberg DM, DeLand F, Kim E, et al: Use of radiolabeled antibodies to carcinoembryonic antigens for the detection and localization of diverse cancers by external photoscanning. N Engl J Med 298:1384, 1978.
6. Goldenberg DM, Kim EE, DeLand FH, et al: Clinical radioimmunodetection of cancer with radioactive antibodies to human chorionic gonadotropin. Science 208:1284, 1980.
7. Belitsky P, Ghoset T, Aquino J, et al: Radionuclide imaging of primary renal-cell carcinoma by I-131-labeled antitumor antibody. J Nucl Med 19:427, 1978.
8. Levine G, Ballou B, Reiland J, et al: Localization of I-131-labeled tumor-specific monoclonal antibody in the tumor-bearing BALB/c mouse. J Nucl Med 21:570, 1980.
9. Goldenberg DM: Radioimmunodetection of cancer workshop. Cancer Res 40:2957, 1980.
10. Wright T, Sinanan M, Harrington D, et al: Immunoglobin: Applications to scanning and treatment. Appl Rad 8:120, 1979.
11. Brown DH, Byrd BL, Carlton JE, et al: A quantitative study of the subcellular localization of ^{67}Ga. Cancer Res 36:956, 1976.
12. Hoffer PB, Huberty JP, Khayam-Bashi H: The association of ^{67}Ga and lactoferrin. J Nucl Med 18:713, 1977.
13. Woolfenden JM, Nevin WS, Barber HB, et al: Bronchoscopic tumor detection using a miniature radiation detector and cobalt-57 bleomycin. J Nucl Med 21:P33, 1980.
14. Som P, Atkins HL, Bandoypadhyay D, et al: A fluorinated glucose analog, 2-fluoro-2-deoxy-D-glucose (F-18): Nontoxic tracer for rapid tumor detection. J Nucl Med 21:670, 1980.
15. Rousseau J, Autenrieth D, van Lier JE: Technetium-99m tetrasulfophthalocyanine as a potential tumor scanning agent. J Nucl Med 21-P37, 1980.

16. Reske SN, Vyska K, Reske K, et al: I-131 DNase, a potential tumor imaging agent. J Nucl Med 21:P36, 1980.
17. Kuhl DE, Edwards RQ: Image separation radioisotope scanning. Radiology 80:653, 1963.
18. Kuhl DE, Edwards RQ, Ricci AR, et al: The Mark IV system for radionuclide computed tomography of the brain. Radiology 121:405, 1976.
19. Anger HO: Tomographic gamma-ray scanner with simultaneous readout of several planes, in Gottschalk A, Beck RN (eds): Fundamental Problems in Scanning. Springfield, Ill, C C Thomas, 1968, p 195.
20. Hauser MF, Gottschalk A: Comparison of the Anger tomographic scanner and the 15 inch scintillation camera in gallium imaging. J Nucl Med 18:603, 1978.
21. Phelps ME: Emission computed tomography. Semin Nucl Med 8:337, 1977.
22. Galaska CSB, Doyle FH: The response to therapy of skeletal metastasis from mammary cancer. Br J Surg 59:7, 1972.
23. Corcoran RJ, Thrall JH, Kyle RN, et al: Solitary abnormalities in bone scans of patients with extra-osseous malignancies. Radiology 121:663, 1976.
24. Sullivan DC, Taylor JW, Gottschalk A: The use of ultrasound to enhance the diagnostic utility of the equivocal liver scintigraph. J Nucl Med 18:621, 1977.
25. Tonami N, Hisada K: ^{201}Tl scintigraphy in postoperative detection of thyroid cancer: A comparative study. Radiology 136:461, 1980.
26. Brown JP, Wright PW, Hart CE, et al: Protein antigens of normal and malignant human cells identified by immunoprecipitation with monoclonal antibodies. J Biol Chem 255:4980, 1980.

FIVE

Vascular and Interventional Radiology

Franklin J. Miller

BACKGROUND AND INTRODUCTION

Diagnostic arteriography at present plays a relatively minor role in the detection, but a larger role in the preoperative assessment, of many solid tumors. These tumors include those of the head and neck, retroperitoneum, abdomen, pelvis, and extremities.

Although few advances have been made recently in angiography in terms of increasing diagnostic accuracy, its use is often necessary to define the extent of tumor and for mapping vascular fields preoperatively. With the continuing improvement in imaging potential associated with the newer technologies, such as ultrasound and computed tomography (CT), the role of diagnostic angiography will continue to diminish. This trend is illustrated by the significant decline in utilization of diagnostic angiography in the work-up of the patient suspected of having a cerebral mass lesion. In most institutions, an enhanced CT scan forms the first screening procedure and almost invariably proves to be sensitive in the detection of the mass lesion. Consequently, angiographic volume in such settings has decreased by 20 to 30 percent. Cerebral arteriography is still performed in many instances of intracerebral mass lesions prior to any definitive surgical treatment.

Selective intra-arterial perfusion of tumors through percutaneously placed catheters has proven effective in the palliation of a number of cancers, particularly those within the liver. Technical difficulties and complications have precluded more widespread application of this palliative approach, as has the shortage of adequately trained medical person-

49

nel, all of which will be discussed under research recommendations. In some instances, bulky vascular tumors can be embolized with occlusive devices or inert foreign material, either preoperatively or for the palliation of local symptoms or distant metastatic disease.

STATE OF THE ART

State of the Art in Diagnosis

Head and Neck.   Cerebral arteriography will be employed in many instances of suspected intracranial neoplasms even when the diagnosis is evident by computed tomography. This study allows the surgeon both the advantage of a vascular road map and the opportunity to more accurately stage the patient. Arteriography is usually not necessary with multiple metastatic lesions, intrasellar lesions without parasellar or suprasellar extension, and in patients who are inoperable for other reasons.

Extracerebral lesions such as juvenile angiofibromas, glomus jugulare tumors, and uncommon lesions at the base of the skull (such as chordomas) will require arteriography for preoperative assessment even when the diagnosis is evident by other clinical and radiographic techniques, since these tumors lie adjacent to either the carotid arteries or the jugular veins.

Thorax.   Arteriography has a limited role in the diagnosis and staging of neoplasms of the thorax, except in the uncommon instance of intracardiac lesions.

The detection and staging of pulmonary neoplasms will continue to be made by routine radiographic techniques and computed tomography. Bronchial arteriography and pulmonary arteriography are rarely indicated in the staging of primary lung cancers.

Cardiac tumors, including atrial myxomas, are studied best by ultrasound and angiography preoperatively. Right atrial, right ventricular, and left ventricular injections will allow detection of tumors in those respective chambers, whereas a pulmonary arteriogram will safely define left atrial myxomas. Coronary arteriography for these cardiac tumors may be helpful when the other studies are equivocal or additional preoperative information is necessary.

Abdomen

LIVER. For the diagnosis of primary or metastatic liver disease, the nuclide scan remains a well established examination with an accuracy of approximately 95 percent in detecting liver tumors greater than 2 cm in size. Nuclide scanning is by its nature a sensitive examination but is not specific in separating cystic from solid lesions. When the nuclide study is equivocal, the addition of ultrasound will increase diagnostic accuracy significantly. Computed tomography is indicated where expertise in ultrasound is not available or nuclide scanning is indeterminate. CT and radionuclide liver screening share approximately equal detection efficiencies.[1,2]

Arteriography will remain indicated as a diagnostic examination prior to resection of solitary lesions within the liver, whether the lesion is a hepatoma or a solitary metastatic lesion. Arteriography will on occasion be necessary to distinguish cancer from multiple hemangiomas in the adult liver when computed tomography is indeterminant.

PANCREAS. Approximately 19,000 patients die every year in the United States from carcinoma of the pancreas, an overall incidence of approximately 25 deaths per 100,000 population. This rate increases to 50 per 100,000 for white men in the United States. Although several reviews suggest an increasing incidence of carcinoma of the pancreas,[3,4] the higher incidence may be the result of an increase in detection efficiency. Little, if any, improvement has been made in the outcome of this disease. The present state of the art of CT scanning should allow for detection of mass lesions in the pancreas of approximately 2 cm in size, but there is no evidence that this will change the survival statistics. At the present time, surgical resection of small lesions remains the only hope for survival in a patient with carcinoma of the pancreas. On rare occasions, ultrasound and CT of the pancreas may be normal, but the clinical suspicion of cancer is high; in those instances arteriography should be used for diagnostic purposes. Percutaneous pancreatic aspiration for cytologic diagnosis has significant diagnostic potential but is underutilized in the United States, primarily because insufficient numbers of trained personnel are available for cytologic interpretation, and, to a lesser extent, there are insufficient numbers of personnel trained in aspiration techniques.

Laparotomy for the purpose of diagnosis of carcinoma of the pancreas where surgery is not needed for gastrointestinal bypass is no longer necessary where aspiration techniques are available. Successful aspiration biopsies of the pancreas without complications, utilizing the thin needle technique (Chiba), have been reported.[5,23] Obviously, this technique can save considerable patient morbidity, mortality, and cost.[6]

KIDNEYS AND ADRENAL GLANDS. The approach to suspected renal carcinoma is best made by an intravenous urogram, followed by an ultrasound to further characterize the mass lesion. Arteriography is usually performed preoperatively in large, bulky tumors along with evaluation of the inferior vena cava. CT currently plays a lesser diagnostic role with renal mass lesions because of the accuracy of ultrasound, but CT does play an important staging role.

Significant progress has recently been made in the study of adrenal glands by CT. Small mass lesions within the adrenal gland were previously studied by venography, which is very accurate. Newer CT units can detect small (1 cm) nodules, although these tumors are usually benign and prove to be adenomas. When an adrenal carcinoma presents as an obvious mass lesion, it can be readily identified on a urogram. Arteriography usually reveals a relatively vascular mass. CT is often performed to identify the local extent of the tumor. Angiography is used more for preoperative staging of these large adrenal cancers, whereas CT is the preferred diagnostic method. Hormone assay of adrenal vein samples is more useful in benign lesions of the adrenal gland than in carcinomas.

RETROPERITONEAL STRUCTURES, EXCLUDING THE KIDNEY AND ADRENAL GLANDS. Until the advent of CT scanning, arteriography was the primary method for detection or confirmation of retroperitoneal tumors. Currently, computed tomography is the best modality for study of this area. A role for arteriography, however, remains for preoperative staging of some retroperitoneal tumors.

PELVIS. Arteriography plays only a supplemental role in the definition and staging of large, bulky tumors prior to surgical removal. Ultrasound and CT play a greater role than arteriography at the present time.

EXTREMITIES. The use of arteriography in the diagnosis of soft tissue tumors of the extremities or bone tumors has virtually disappeared. Standard tomography and CT can more accurately define tumor extent and aid in treatment planning. Arteriography is occasionally helpful in soft tissue tumors.[7–10]

State of the Art: Therapeutic Considerations

Whereas the use of arteriography for diagnostic purposes plays a smaller role than it did 10 years ago, the role of interventional angiographic procedures in the treatment of cancer is increasing. Currently, interventional angiographic techniques are used for preoperative devascularization of tumors. Embolization has also been used for palliation of bone pain from a variety of lesions.[11] Perfusion of chemotherapeutic agents into the liver has been shown to be helpful in selected patients with metastatic disease.[17]

Head and Neck. It has recently been shown that it is feasible to embolize certain materials into the intracerebral circulation.[12–14] To date, embolic materials have been successfully used in the treatment of arteriovenous malformations and could be used in the treatment of a selected few inoperable brain tumors. These techniques have also been applied to the devascularization of tumors of the head and neck to help decrease operative blood loss.

The application of intra-arterial perfusion of brain tumors has been effected without complications.[15] Only future controlled trials will define the safety and usefulness of this difficult procedure.

Thorax. Bronchial artery catheterization has been utilized to infuse lung tumors. Some dramatic responses of adenocarcinomas following infusion with mitamycin-C have been noted.[10] This technique is technically difficult and not without hazard, since the spinal cord may be supplied by branches of the same bronchial arteries. Also, metastatic lesions may not be perfused by the same arteries which supply the primary tumor.

Liver. Intra-arterial perfusion of 5-fluorouracil has been reported to be less hazardous and more effective than systemic infusion of the same drug.[17] Currently, this technique is being used in selected patients with bladder, colon, and breast cancer with a decrease in morbidity, and one study suggests a 4 to 6 month prolongation of life.[21] As other chemotherapeutic agents are developed, they should be evaluated in controlled trials.

Hepatic artery ligation for tumor palliation has been performed in the past. However, rapid collaterals to the liver develop following ligation. Percutaneous catheter techniques can be used to embolize the distal or proximal hepatic arteries. One recent report shows that the use of Gelfoam® plugs followed by coils placed into the hepatic artery can be tolerated by patients with metastatic disease.[22]

Pancreas and Bile Ducts. Intra-arterial therapy for pancreatic carcinoma has been implemented without complications in two patients using embolization techniques with deposition of radioactive yttrium simultaneously.[18]

Kidneys and Adrenal Glands. Currently, at the M.D. Anderson Hospital and Tumor Institute, many hypernephromas over 5 cm are preoperatively treated with embolization techniques. This procedure seems to make the surgery technically easier and results in less blood loss. This technique has not been universally employed because some urologists believe that most renal tumors can be handled adequately without this preoperative interventional procedure. This same group has reported on 100 patients with hypernephromas whose tumors were embolized prior to surgery. Of 50 patients with lung metastases, 6 showed complete disappearance of their metastases with preoperative embolization and Provera with a 1 year follow-up. Five patients showed partial regression and 14 were stable. The courses of 25 patients were unchanged. Although it is premature to look at the survival statistics on these patients, no other similar consecutive series of 50 hypernephroma patients exists in which metastatic lung lesions decreased in size in 50 percent of the patients and these patients survived 1 year.[19]

LIMITATIONS OF CURRENT TECHNIQUES

Diagnostic Limitations
Angiography is currently limited to detection of tumors of approximately 2 cm in size or more within the abdomen or pelvis, unless they are very vascular.

Aspiration biopsy techniques have also found limited application. There are several factors responsible for this. First, few radiologists are trained to do biopsy procedures. Second, a lack of understanding and skepticism in referring clinicians exists as to the value of this technique. Third, limited numbers of personnel in cytologic interpretation are available. Without expert cytologic interpretation, the use of aspiration techniques for biopsy of the pancreas, lung, nodes, or other mass lesions is not indicated.

Therapeutic Limitations
Currently, one of the uses of therapeutic techniques in angiography is the perfusion of metastatic liver disease (usually colonic primaries) with 5-fluorouracil and other chemotherapeutic agents. The technique is limited in that frequently there is difficulty in entering the proper hepatic artery selectively and infusion of the stomach via the gastroduodenal artery, causing gastrointestinal upset in the patient. New techniques with flotation balloons may solve this problem. Care of the perfusion catheters is often a problem but can be accomplished at home in some instances. Lack of experience in doing subselective catheterization and the time required for the procedures are some of the current limitations in expanding the use of perfusion of metastatic liver disease outside of large medical centers. Acceptance of this procedure is also limited because of the lack of any well established, controlled series showing prolongation of life.

Certainly, perfusion of brain lesions requires expertise, and catheter care is of utmost importance in preventing thrombosis or clot formation. These techniques are possible, but few physicians are experienced in their application.

New embolization materials are necessarily limited because of FDA guidelines. A few individuals currently have FDA approval for investigation of silicone rubber, a valuable embolic compound. A few other investigators have approval for use of acrylate materials (rapid occlusive agent in the blood), but approval of this product requires long-term, costly studies to establish safety.[20]

Pulmonary and Mediastinal Tumors. The vessels supplying mediastinal and pulmonary tumors are complex and frequently difficult to catheterize, making infusion or occlusion therapy in these patients less promising.

Liver. Although frequently difficult and time-consuming, hepatic artery catheterization is possible for perfusion of liver neoplasms. Catheter care is vitally important but can be taught to the average individual and family, allowing outpatient management in some instances.

Intra-arterial perfusion has historically been looked on with disfavor, but the view on intensive catheter perfusion for colon cancer metastatic to the liver seems to be more optimistic.[17,21,22]

Pancreas. The limitations of treating the pancreas by angiographic techniques are strictly mechanical. Techniques are now available in which flotation balloons are used to enter small vessels. In selected cases, the catheter can be placed at the origin of at least one neoplastic vessel supplying a pancreatic tumor, and can subsequently be used for therapy with drugs, occlusive therapy, deposition of radioactive compounds, or a combination of all three.

Kidneys. Preoperative occlusion of large renal tumors has found application in only a few major centers. When performed, pain and fever are not uncommon and can be expected to last 2 to 3 days, often requiring narcotics for control.

Retroperitoneum. The anatomic barriers to intra-arterial therapy for retroperitoneal tumors include the multiple arterial feeders from the aorta and the hypovascular nature of many of these tumors. These problems preclude application of this therapeutic approach in most instances.

RECOMMENDATIONS FOR RESEARCH SUPPORT

Improved Materials for Interventional Radiology
Technical limitations often frustrate the successful application of interventional radiologic techniques. Research support is needed to address these issues, as follows.

Balloon Catheter Technology. Current problems with small balloon catheters include the lack of an easy delivery system through a large outer catheter, a high coefficient of friction between the outer and inner catheters, and the lack of reliable mechanisms for balloon detachment. It would be desirable to develop a reliable detachable and nondetachable balloon of small diameter (0.038 inches) uninflated.

RECOMMENDATION. An ad hoc committee of individuals from private industry and the radiologic community needs to be formed to provide direction in solving the complex technical problems summarized above.

Priority: 1
Duration: 1 to 3 years
Probability of Success: high

The Development and Testing of Injectable Intravascular Occlusive Materials. There have been few well organized studies of the chemical, physical, and safety features of the currently utilized intravascular occlusive agents. New and safer agents need to be developed which can be more easily utilized.

It is recommended that a safe, intravascular group of thrombotic agents be developed which can be delivered easily through a 0.038 inch balloon catheter.

Priority: 2
Duration: 3 years
Probability of Success: high

Research Recommendations: Organ Systems

Metastatic Cancer to the Liver. Metastatic disease to the liver most frequently occurs from a primary gastrointestinal site, usually the colon. This remains a difficult treatment problem. Infusion of chemotherapeutic agents has been tried and has shown evidence of palliation, but only equivocal evidence for prolonged survival. Poorly controlled studies have led to general skepticism among clinicians as to the potential role of infusion therapy.

RECOMMENDATION. Support should be provided for a controlled, national, multicenter trial in the study of intravascular perfusion of metastatic colon cancer to the liver.

Priority: 2
Duration: 4 years
Probability of Success: excellent

Pancreatic Carcinoma. As mentioned above, little progress in prolonging survival of patients with pancreatic carcinoma has occurred. Some promise has been shown subsequent to radiation therapy; however, no controlled trial has been developed to evaluate the role of interventional angiography or perfusion techniques with these tumors.

RECOMMENDATION. A multicenter evaluation is recommended to assess the use of biodegradable starch microspheres used alone or in combination with chemotherapeutic drugs in pancreatic cancer. A second controlled trial should assess the utilization of radioactive materials attached or tagged to embolic substances and then delivered to the pancreatic tumor site via flow-directed (balloon) catheters.

Priority: 2
Duration: 4 years
Probability of Success: moderate

Hypernephroma. As noted above, it is not uncommon to encounter difficulty in the control of both local and metastatic renal cancer. The initial experience at M.D. Anderson Hospital and Tumor Clinic justifies further evaluation of the role of interventional angiography in both the preoperative management and the definitive treatment of the inoperable renal tumor patient.

RECOMMENDATION. A multicenter trial should be developed to evaluate the preoperative embolization of primary renal tumors which are large and vascular. A second, more complex, larger trial should be implemented to evaluate the role of embolization of the primary, inoperable renal tumor in patients with metastatic disease. An immune response is suggested to explain the regression of the metastatic lesions. All facets of this problem need evaluation through a large, multicenter protocol including immunologists, urologists, and radiologists.

Priority: 1
Duration: 5 years
Probability of Success: moderate

Primary Intracerebral Tumors and Brain Metastases. The failure of conventional, surgical, and external radiation therapy techniques to control both primary and metastatic brain tumors is well known. In certain instances, these tumors are assessable to occlusive vascular procedures and perfusion techniques.

RECOMMENDATION. Clinical trials should be developed to evaluate the impact of catheter embolization and perfusion of primary and metastatic cerebral tumors. Obviously, controlled trials would not be appropriate in this setting. The patient population would necessarily be limited initially to those individuals with unfavorable and inoperable tumors.

Priority: 3
Duration: 4 years
Probability of Success: fair

Research Training and Clinician Education

Many clinicians, even those found within major medical centers, are unaware of the potential applications of interventional angiographic techniques. Similarly, there is an even more serious deficiency in the availability of trained radiologic and pathologic personnel to join forces in the application of aspiration biopsy techniques.

RECOMMENDATION. It is recommended that funding be made available for postgraduate training of cytologic personnel and radiologists in the application of these biopsy techniques. This training should be performed in acknowledged centers of excellence. In addition, programmed educational materials should be made available to both orient and reinforce the educational programs. Finally, medical school curricula should include references to these techniques.

ACKNOWLEDGMENTS

I would like to thank Drs. P. Ruben Koehler and D. Edward Mineau for their constructive remarks.

REFERENCES

1. Bryan PJ, et al: Correlation of computed tomography, gray scale ultrasonography, and radionuclide imaging of the liver in detecting space-occupying processes. Radiology 124:387–393, 1977.

2. MacCarty RL, et al: Retrospective comparison of radionuclide scans and computed tomography of the liver and pancreas. AJR 129:23–28, 1977.
3. Krain LS, et al: The rising incidence of carcinoma of the pancreas—real or apparent. J Surg Oncol 2:115–124, 1970.
4. Benarde MA, et al: A cohort analysis of pancreatic cancer. Cancer 39:2160–2163, 1977.
5. Christoffersen P, et al: Preoperative pancreas aspiration biopsies. Acta Pathol Microbiol Scand (suppl) 212:28–32, 1970.
6. Haaga JR, et al: CT guided biopsy. Cleve Clin Q 44(1): 27–33, 1977.
7. Levin DC, et al: Arteriography of peripheral hemangiomas. Radiology 121:625–630, 1976.
8. Levin DC, et al: Arteriography in diagnosis and management of acquired peripheral soft-tissue masses. Radiology 103:53–58, 1972.
9. Volgeli E: Arteriography in bone tumors. Skeletal Radiol 1:3–14, 1976.
10. Weinberger G, et al: Computed tomography in the evaluation of sarcomatous tumors of the thigh. AJR 130:115–118, 1978.
11. Wallace S, et al: Arterial occlusion of pelvic bone tumors. Cancer 43:322–328, 1979.
12. Hilal SK, et al: Therapeutic percutaneous embolization for extra-axial vascular lesions of the head, neck and spine. J Neurosurg 43:275–287, 1975.
13. Kerber C: Balloon catheter with a calibrated leak. Radiology 120:547–550, 1976.
14. Pevsner PH: Micro-balloon catheter for superselective angiography and therapeutic occlusion. AJR 128:225–230, 1977.
15. Pevsner P: Personal communication 1978.
16. Boijsen E: Personal communication 1979.
17. Ansfield FJ, et al: Further clinical studies with intrahepatic arterial infusion with 5-fluorouracil. Cancer 36:2413–2417, 1976.
18. Eisenberg H: Personal communication 1981.
19. Chuang V, et al: Experience in 100 renal carcinoma infarctions. Paper 245 presented at the 65th Scientific Assembly and Annual Meeting of the Radiologic Society of North America, Atlanta, Georgia, December 1979.
20. Page RC, et al: Chronic toxicity studies of methyl-2-cyanoacrylate in dogs and rats, in proceedings of the Symposium on Physiologic Adhesives. Houston, Tex, University of Texas Graduate School, 1966.
21. Chuang VP, et al: Hepatic arterial redistribution for intraarterial infusion of hepatic neoplasms. Radiology 135:295–299, 1980.
22. Chuang VP, et al: Current status of transcatheter management of neoplasms. Cardiovasc Interventional Radiol 3:256–265, 1980.
23. Zornoza J: Abdomen, in Zornoza J: Percutaneous Needle Biopsy. Baltimore, Williams & Wilkins, 1981, pp 102–140.

SIX

Head and Neck Tumors

Robert E. Anderson and Lee F. Rogers

The diagnosis and management of tumors of the head and neck concerns many specialty areas in medicine, including the neurosciences (neurosurgery, neurology, neuroradiology, neuro-ophthalmology, etc.), ENT, and the subspecialties of chemotherapy and radiation oncology. For purposes of this review of imaging methods for tumors of the head and neck, anatomic areas will be divided into those which fall within the traditional boundaries of neuroradiology and those which are more often dealt with by other subspecialty areas of radiology.

Historically, plain film examination, tomography, nuclear medicine, and angiography have been the mainstays in head and neck tumor diagnosis. Recently, computed tomography has emerged as the most powerful imaging tool in the cranial cavity, orbit, and most deep facial structures. Further research may disclose broadened roles for positron emission tomography (PET), computer-enhanced ultrasound and radiography, and nuclear magnetic resonance imaging.

STATE OF THE ART

Neuroradiologic Techniques
The cranial cavity and facial structure (paranasal sinuses, nasal cavity, and orbits) may be grouped together at this point, since most current neuroradiologic methods have a similar yield in these anatomic zones.

Examination of the head, including facial structures, may be carried out at the present time via the following conventional means: plain film radiography, computed tomography, cerebral angiography, and pneumoencephalography.

Plain film radiography remains a valuable technique in many categories of disease of the face and cranial cavity. Unfortunately, the number of tumors visible on plain films is relatively small. For example, most intracranial neoplasms show no abnormality on plain film examinations. Tumors of the facial structures become apparent as they displace air in sinus cavities, etc., but are not recognized as neoplastic until bone destruction is evident. Soft tissue tumors in the neck are generally not detectable on plain film examination until very large.

Computed tomography (CT) has had a major impact on the diagnosis of disease states in all portions of the cranial cavity and face.[1-6] It has proven to be the most accurate means of intracranial tumor detection.[7] The efficacy of cranial CT is elegantly documented by the declining volume of diagnostic angiograms, pneumoencephalograms, and isotope brain scans in institutions where CT is established.[8]

Unfortunately, the initial impression that CT scanning would be a completely noninvasive test was incorrect. A high false negative detection rate was noted in early series due to the isodense nature of some metastases, gliomas, and meningiomas.[9] Aqueous iodinated contrast materials must be infused prior to scanning for tumor detection. Plain CT scans are generally not required prior to enhanced scans, since virtually all neoplasms are evident after intravenous contrast agents are infused.[10]

Cerebral angiography remains a useful study in examining patients suspected of having malignant lesions in the cranial cavity and face. While less accurate than CT scanning for tumor detection, cerebral angiography frequently supplies valuable information regarding the nature of the lesion and its blood supply preoperatively. For example, the angiographic confirmation of a middle meningeal arterial supply and a homogenous tumor stain are virtually diagnostic of meningioma. Occlusion of an arterial branch is very rarely seen with tumors and supports a diagnosis of stroke. Similarly, a vascular malformation may occasionally mimic a neoplasm on CT, while its true nature is usually obvious on angiograms.

Pneumoencephalography is presently rarely used in intracranial tumor detection where modern CT facilities are available. In the preoperative management of a patient with a pituitary mass lesion, pneumoencephalography may still assist in recognizing the cephalic extent of the lesion into the suprasellar cistern. Similarly, parasellar air serves as a useful reference point during transsphenoidal sellar surgery utilizing fluoroscopic guidance.

The Oral Cavity, Salivary Glands, Larynx and Hypopharynx, and Thyroid

Oral Cavity. Plain film radiography, including special "panoramic" views of the mandible and alveolar ridge of the maxilla area, is utilized to determine the presence or absence of direct extension of tumors of the gingiva floor, mouth, tongue, and hard palate.

Salivary Glands. Sialography is frequently employed in the evaluation of salivary gland tumors. However, imaging techniques play a small role in the initial detection of these tumors.

Larynx and Hypopharynx. Plain film radiography (more specifically, the soft tissue lateral view of the neck), tomography, barium swallow, laryngography, and xerographic examinations obtained in the lateral projection are frequently utilized in the pretreatment staging of a patient with a laryngeal tumor. Computed tomography of the larynx and pharynx has recently been shown to be useful in tumor assessment and is probably the best radiographic tool in evaluating primary laryngeal tumors at the present time.[11-16]

The goals of imaging in a patient with a known laryngeal primary tumor are to assist in staging the patient, complementing both clinical and endoscopic examination. Such studies should particularly be concerned with mobility of the vocal cords, subglottic extension, and cartilaginous invasion. Current generation CT scanning can most easily accomplish these goals at the present.[17]

Thyroid. Nuclear scintigraphy and ultrasound are the most frequently employed thyroid imaging techniques utilized today. Little experience with CT evaluation of the thyroid, together with resolution limitations, have restricted the application of this technique.

Nuclear imaging of the thyroid has been the traditional first imaging choice in the evaluation of the clinically palpable thyroid nodule. At the present time, many centers recommend as a more appropriate first choice to determine whether the lesion is cystic or solid. If the lesion is cystic, percutaneous aspiration is possible, with subsequent laboratory analysis of the fluid content.

If the lesion is solid, radionuclide scanning should subsequently be utilized to determine whether the lesion is functional or not, with functional nodules being significantly less likely to harbor carcinomas.

Controversy exists as to the proper mode of evaluating the individual who has had prior irradiation of the head and neck. Since many of the subsequent tumors noted in these patients are either multifocal or arise in areas other than the clinically palpable abnormality, both physical examination and scan images of the thyroid play a complimentary role.[18]

LIMITATIONS OF CURRENT TECHNIQUES

Standard Neuroradiologic Techniques

Plain film study of the head and neck is severely limited by the inability to visualize most neoplasms in this part of the anatomy with this technique. Few intracranial tumors have plain film findings. Meningiomas, growing near a calvarial margin, may exhibit dramatic skull film abnormalities, but the majority are radiographically occult. A small percentage of astrocytomas may calcify, but even with CT evaluation, this characteristic is more helpful in a differential setting than in providing a detection advantage. Many, if not a majority, of face, oral, and pharyngeal regions show no plain film findings until advanced disease is present. Digitized methods for plain film examination (computed radiology) may improve the situation slightly, but early experience indicates a limited role for computed radiology in craniofacial tumor detection.

Computed tomography is the single most effective neuroradiologic tool available for the diagnosis of lesions within the cranial cavity, facial skeleton, and portions of the soft tissues of the neck. Recent improvements in spatial resolution, shortened scan input times, and more experience with contrast enhancement techniques have improved the accuracy of this method greatly over the last 5 years. Current limitations of the CT method include inability to see most lesions under 1 cm in size and inability to detect those tumors showing no x-ray absorption difference from the surrounding normal tissues.

Cerebral angiography remains a valuable method of tumor evaluation. Diagnostic angiography is infrequently utilized in tumor diagnosis at present for reasons of detection efficiency, cost, and morbidity.

Angiography is, however, frequently useful in defining the blood supply of a known mass lesion. However, tumors of the orbit, paranasal sinuses, and oral cavity and most soft tissue cancers of the neck exhibit very little abnormal vascular supply on angiographic examination.

In institutions with modern CT scanning capabilities, pneumoencephalography is seldom used. Similarly, the standard radionuclide brain scan has no current role in intracranial tumor detection, where high quality CT scans are available.

Positron emission tomography and nuclear magnetic resonance imaging have a major potential role in central nervous system (CNS) tumor evaluation and are described in detail in another chapter.

Developments in computer-enhanced ultrasound imaging of head and neck masses have been limited mainly to the soft tissues of the neck thus far. Computer enhancement of radiographic and fluoroscopic images (CR and CF) may provide images of the head and neck which are superior to film radiography for certain applications, but it is doubtful that these techniques will have much impact on tumor detection.

The Oral Cavity, Salivary Glands, Larynx and Hypopharynx, and Thyroid

Oral Cavity. Inspection and palpation are quite adequate for early tumor detection in this region. Current radiographic methods would appear to be satisfactory for the detection of extension of oral malignancies to surrounding bone when gross invasion of local osseous structures has occurred.[12]

Salivary Glands. Sialography is not universally utilized in the evaluation of salivary gland tumors. Its use does allow localization of tumors when small, but does not give an indication of their malignant or benign characteristics. Computed tomography has only been utilized to a limited extent in the evaluation of salivary tumors, and the impact of this technique on tumor staging is not known as yet.

Larynx and Hypopharynx. The combination of plain film radiography, xerography, laryngography, and CT provides excellent imaging means to delineate the extent of tumors in this area.[16] Laryngography has been infrequently applied in the staging work-up of laryngeal tumors, often due to lack of experience with the technique. New generation rapid scanning CT probably will replace the need for staging laryngograms in most centers where this equipment is available.

Thyroid. Nuclear imaging of the thyroid is size- and location-dependent but provides the additional information concerning the functional status of a nodule. Since functioning nodules are rarely malignant, these lesions are then treated medically.

Ultrasound with currently improving resolution is increasingly used to determine the nature of a thyroid nodule. Furthermore, aspiration of cystic lesions makes this technique even more specific.[18]

Resolution remains the common problem limiting the sensitivity of both ultrasound and radionuclide scintigraphy. Refinements are needed in both scanning techniques, together with broader application of percutaneous biopsy for the newly detected nodules.

RECOMMENDATIONS FOR RESEARCH SUPPORT

Most imaging techniques for head and neck tumors are limited by imaging equipment factors to varying degrees. Therefore, many of the recommendations for research support which follow are equipment-related. While equipment manufacturers have been responsible for many advances in equipment design, it is appropriate that design improvements also be funded through research grants. Numerous design improvements which seem to represent obvious advances in diagnostic methods are not being developed and may not be forthcoming unless evaluated in a research setting and shown to be of practical significance.

Improvements in Imaging Systems

Computed Tomography. While current computed tomography equipment is capable of detecting a high percentage of intracranial and facial neoplasms, a number of areas for research exist which may yield important further advances in CT techniques. These areas include at least the following.

FURTHER EVALUATION OF MONOCHROMATIC OR DUAL-ENERGY X-RAY SOURCES FOR CT SCANNERS. Evidence suggests that selective absorption of different constituents of soft tissues may produce data more specific for different kinds of lesions than is presently possible. At the present time, many categories of pathology—including primary brain tumors, secondary brain tumors, cerebral infarction, trauma, viral and bacterial infection, radiation, and drug damage—cause similar CT scan appearances. A major improvement in the use of CT scans in tumor detections and management would result from improved specificity of the CT scan data.[19–21]

BETTER CT DISPLAY SYSTEMS. Data are available which suggest that the standard CT TV screen display format does not match the viewer's visual system particularly well. Improved display systems may make small tumors easier to see.[22,23] Three-dimensional displays of multiple CT images will also aid in interpretation of scan images by providing the viewing physician with a more realistic representation of the anatomy being studied.[24]

INFUSION OF INTRAVENOUS CONTRAST MATERIAL. While infusion of intravenous contrast material may enhance the visibility of an abnormality on CT scan, studies are being done which indicate that the manner in which the contrast material is infused does make a difference in lesion detection.[25-29] Studies of different chemical substances for contrast enhancement of neoplasms may also result in improved tumor visualization.

CT-GUIDED STEREOTAXIC BIOPSY PROCEDURES. These procedures are beginning to emerge as safer, more accurate techniques in obtaining tissue from deep cerebral lesions.[30] Further refinements are needed in these biopsy techniques. Therapeutic applications—such as precise implantation of radioactive sources and direct infusion of chemotherapeutic agents into brain lesions—should also be explored further.

Priority: 1
Duration: 1 to 5 years
Probability of Success: high

Ultrasound. Examination of the cranial contents beyond infancy is not feasible at present due to the formidable barrier to ultrasound presented by mature bone.[31] Experimental work is under way in which computer enhancement techniques are being used to reconstruct weak signals coming back from intracranial contents through the intact adult skull. These efforts should be encouraged.

Soft tissues of the neck are more suitable for ultrasonic investigation. Thyroid ultrasound scans have proven of value. Further work in defining typical echo patterns ("tissue signatures") may yield more specific ultrasonic data regarding the nature of a thyroid mass or other soft tissue mass in the neck prior to biopsy. Further basic work in defining the echo patterns from different normal and abnormal soft tissues should be pursued.

Priority: 1
Duration: 3 to 5 years
Probability of Success: moderate

Computed Tomography-related Efficacy Studies

The value of CT methods in the detection of brain tumors has been adequately demonstrated. Cost-effectiveness studies of various kinds seem to indicate that CT scanning is a cost-effective method in the head and neck. At least two important aspects of CT scanner utilization, however, have not been adequately addressed.

The Proper Application of CT and Other Radiologic Tests for Various Symptom Complexes. The appropriate choice of various radiologic tests in the detection and staging of head and neck tumors is confusing to many clinicians *and* radiologists at present. Various "decision trees" for the proper application of the various radiologic modalities are now being introduced.[32] While it may be possible to agree upon the proper sequence of radiologic tests for the evaluation of a given symptom complex, these decision trees have not been tested from a cost-effectiveness standpoint. A large, multi-institutional study should be planned in which standardized approaches to a variety of common symptom complexes are examined not only for efficiency in detecting disease states, but also for the cost-effectiveness of the various "algorithms." For example, a nuclear medicine brain scan may have an 85 percent chance of showing the presence of an abnormality but not be cost-effective if a CT scan is still deemed essential in the work-up of the patient.

Priority: 2
Duration: 3 to 5 years
Probability of Success: high

Cost versus Effectiveness of CT Scanners. Another type of cost-effectiveness study regarding computed tomography equipment is urgently needed at the present time. There is no question that CT scanning of the head and neck provides extremely valuable information in both the detection and management of neoplasms. It is also obvious that not every hospital or other health facility which might wish to have a modern CT unit can justify the installation of such a sophisticated unit, which may cost as much as $1,000,000 to install and several hundred thousand dollars annually to operate. Experience with CT scanners from the original EMI head scanner to the most sophisticated systems available today leads to the hypothesis that many applications for computed tomography do not require the use of the most sophisticated, expensive CT equipment currently available in the marketplace.

This hypothesis could be tested by well-designed phantom studies in which prototype CT scanner configurations of varying degrees of cost and complexity were studied objectively to determine the size and density characteristics of the smallest lesion each configuration could detect. This information could be used in developing lower-cost CT scanners for use in smaller institutions. Unless objective data are available indicating that lower-cost, simpler CT scanners can be used effectively in tumor detection, such scanners will not be built or marketed.

Priority: 1
Duration: 2 to 3 years
Probability of Success: high

REFERENCES

1. Wende S, Aulich A, Kretzschmar K, et al: Computer tomography in intracranial tumors: Cooperative study of 1958 neoplasms. Radiologe 17:149, 1977.
2. Davis DO: CT in the diagnosis of supratentorial tumors. Semin Roentgenol 12:97, 1977.
3. Momose KJ, New PFJ, Grove AS, et al: The use of computed tomography in ophthalmology. Neuroradiology 15:361, 1975.
4. Wing SD: Direct sagittal scans in computed tomography of the orbits. CT 2:109, 1978.
5. Bernardino ME, Danziger J, Young SE, Wallace S: Computed tomography in ocular neoplastic disease. Am J Roentgenol 131:111, 1978.
6. Hilal SK, Trokel SL: Computerized tomography of the orbit using thin sections. Semin Roentgenol 12:137, 1977.
7. Baker HL, Houser OW, Campbell JK: National Cancer Institute Study: Evaluation of computed tomography in the diagnosis of intracranial neoplasms. Radiology 136:91–96, July 1980.
8. Enlow RA, Hodak JA, Pullen KW: The effect of the computed tomographic scanner on utilization and charges for alternative diagnostic procedures. Radiology 136:413–418, August 1980.
9. New PF, Aronow S, Hesselink JR: National Cancer Institute Study: Evaluation of computed tomography in the diagnosis of intracranial neoplasms. Radiology 136:665–675, September 1980.
10. Potts DG, Abbott GF, von Sneidern JV: National Cancer Institute Study: Evaluation of computed tomography in the diagnosis of intracranial neoplasms: III. Metastatic tumors. Radiology 136:657–664, September 1980.
11. Jing BS: Tumors of the nasopharynx. Radiol Clin North Am 8:323, 1970.
12. Jimenez JR: Roentgen examination of the oropharynx and oral cavity. Radiol Clin North Am 8:413, 1970.
13. Paulus DD Jr, Dodd GD: The roentgen diagnosis of tumors of the nasal cavity and accessory paranasal sinuses. Radiol Clin North Am 8:343, 1970.
14. Wortzman G, Holgate RC: Computerized tomography (CT) in otolaryngology. Laryngoscope 86:1552, 1976.
15. Zimmerman RA, Bilaniuk LT: Computed tomography of sphenoid sinus tumors. CT 1:23, 1977.
16. Jing BS: Roentgen examination of the larynx and hypopharynx. Radiol Clin North Am 8:361, 1970.
17. Mancuso AA, Tamakawa Y, Hanafee WN: CT of the fixed vocal cord. Am J Roentgenol 135:529–534, September 1980.
18. Schneider AB, Pinsky S, Berkerman C, Yun Ryo U: Characteristics of 108 thyroid cancers detected by screening in a population with a history of head and neck irradiation. Cancer 46:1218–1227, 1980.
19. Hounsfield GN: Potential uses of more accurate CT absorption values by filtering. Am J Roentgenol 131:103, 1978.

20. McCullough EC: Factors affecting the use of quantitative information from a CT scanner. Radiology 124:99, 1977.
21. Zatz LM, Alvarez RE: Inaccuracy in computed tomography: Energy dependence of CT values. Radiology 124:91, 1977.
22. Baxter BS, Normann R, Ravindra H: Retinal photoreceptor response and contrast discrimination. Scientific exhibit, SNM, Detroit, June 1980.
23. Baxter BS, Normann R, Knochel J, et al: The role of visual adaptation in diagnostic image interpretation. Work in Progress Presentation for RSNA, Dallas, November 1980.
24. Baxter BS: A 3-D viewing device for interpretation of multiple section images. NCC-80 80:437–440, AFIPS Press, Arlington, VA (Conf. Proc.).
25. Koehler PR, Anderson RE, Baxter BS: The effect of computed tomography viewer controls on anatomical measurements. Radiology 130:189–194, 1979.
26. Wing SD, Anderson RE, Osborn AG: Dynamic cranial computed tomography: Preliminary results. Am J Roentgenol 134:941–943, 1980.
27. Wing SD, Anderson RE, Osborn AG: Cranial computed angiotomography. Presentation at RSNA, Dallas, November 1980.
28. Hayman LA, Evans RA, Hinck VC: Delayed high iodine dose contrast computed tomography. Radiology 136:677–684, September 1980.
29. Shalen PR, Hayman LA, Wallace S, Handel SF: Protocol for delayed contrast enhancement in computed tomography of cerebral neoplasia. Radiology 139:397–402, May 1981.
30. Brown RA, Roberts TS, Osborn AG: Stereotaxic frame and computer software for CT-directed neurosurgical localization. Invest Radiol 15:308–312, July/August 1980.
31. Garrett WJ, Kossoff G, Warran PS: Cerebral ventricular size in children: A two-dimensional ultrasonic study. Radiology 136:711–715, September 1980.
32. Eisenberg R, Amberg J: Algorithmic Approach to Radiology. Mosby & Co., to be published.

SEVEN

Chest Tumors

Anthony V. Proto and Jerome F. Wiot

Bronchogenic carcinoma is the most common malignancy in males and is dramatically increasing in frequency in females.[1] In addition, the lung is a common site of metastatic disease from various primary malignancies. The importance of chest roentgenography is further realized when one considers that chest radiographs account for 30 to 40 percent or more of all examinations performed in general hospital radiology departments. In spite of the frequency of occurrence of chest malignancy, be it primary or secondary, and the frequency of chest radiographic examinations, tumor detection is difficult. Studies have shown that mass lesions can be present for years and are only detected retrospectively.[2]

While many imaging modalities can be used for evaluation and follow-up, it is the initial detection that begins the subsequent evaluation and staging. For early detection to receive the widest application, improvements would be most advantageous if accomplished for the simplest modality, the plain film examination of the chest. Because comparisons must be made, the availability of previous radiographs of similar quality is essential to assess change or detect subtle change.

The need for cost containment must be a consideration with both standard imaging modalities and newer techniques, such as computed tomography (CT). Cost containment must not, however, be in conflict with the realistic goals of early diagnosis. Efficacy studies are necessary to reassess the role of routine lateral chest x-rays, techniques of lung to-

The following have also contributed to this chapter: John D. Armstrong II, M.D.; Stanley Fox, Ph.D.; E. Robert Heitzman, M.D.; Peter Herman, M.D.; Myron Moskowitz, M.D.; Charles Putnam, M.D.; Frederick Stitik, M.D.

71

mography, and CT and its value in the preoperative assessment of the pulmonary nodule.[3]

STATE OF THE ART

Detection of the Lesion

An average primary lung cancer has usually gone through approximately two-thirds to three-quarters of its life cycle before it is detected.[4] Thus detection of the lesion before it has progressed to that point would seemingly result in an increased survival.

The present trend in chest radiography is toward higher kilovoltage techniques (120 to 150 kV). The decrease in contrast and better penetration afforded by these techniques can allow for simultaneous evaluation of the mediastinum and pulmonary parenchyma. Unfortunately, approximately 75 percent of the area of the lung is overlapped by bone,[5] prompting the development of even higher kilovoltage techniques (350 kV). With these techniques, there is a decrease in bony dominance and its distracting effect on the recognition of soft tissue masses in the lung. While mottle and decreased visualization of bony and calcium densities are disadvantages with 350 kV technique, the improved parenchymal and mediastinal penetration may be advantageous in lesion detection.[6] The greater consistency in appearance from one examination to another is also helpful in making comparisons.

The ongoing concern for radiation exposure has brought about the evaluation of film–screen combinations, resulting in decreased patient exposure. The rare-earth screens afford this advantage. Early evaluation seems to indicate that exposure times may be reduced to about one-quarter the times with par speed screens and standard x-ray film.[7] Yet some find objectionable not only the mottle but also the loss in detail on radiographs obtained with current rare-earth film–screen combinations.

Xeroradiographic exposure doses are 7 to 15 times greater than doses with routine film techniques. The advantages of edge enhancement and simultaneous visualization of the mediastinum and lung fields with xeroradiography are thus obtained at a higher radiation cost.[8,9]

Geometric magnification radiography has been shown to demonstrate abnormalities that optical magnification of the routine radiograph may not identify.[10] With magnification radiography, the radiation dose may be three times greater than with routine radiography, if comparable exposure factors are used. However, a total exposure that is less than expected may result.[11] While drawbacks do exist (current equipment capabilities, motion unsharpness, etc.),[10,12] magnification radiography might be of help in detecting pulmonary malignancy. The National Cancer Institute Cooperative Group has indicated in its study of the high risk group of men (those

45 years of age or older who smoke one or more packs of cigarettes per day) that sputum cytology is more sensitive for centrally placed lesions and radiography is more sensitive for peripheral cancers.[13,14] Perhaps magnification radiography may be helpful in localizing these occult central lesions detected with positive sputum cytology.

While bronchography is no longer a common radiographic study, there has been some experience with tantalum bronchography[15,16] and early localization of carcinoma in high risk patients.[17] This technique might also be applicable in localizing the disease if sputum cytology is positive and the chest radiograph is negative.

Finally, recent investigations have indicated that multiple interpretations of the same radiograph can decrease the false negative rate; however, the false positive rate will increase as well. In essence, a trade-off develops and must be evaluated in light of the time involved, cost, and implications for patient care.[18]

Differentiation of Benign from Malignant

On plain film examination, the radiographic distinction between benign and malignant disease is usually difficult. Thus more sophisticated procedures are necessary to allow this distinction.

The classic characteristics searched for in making a radiologic distinction of benign or malignant disease are well known. None, however, are pathognomonic. A mainstay in making such distinction is chest tomography. While coned-down views allow for better detail, full chest tomography to include both lungs and the mediastinum can add information that might not be seen from evaluation of the lesion alone. Currently, multiple tomographic techniques are available.[19] Linear tomography is most widely used, with tomograms being obtained at 1 cm intervals. Pluridirectional motions offer thinner sections for viewing but require additional sections for complete evaluation. Tomograms in oblique and lateral projections are also helpful in assessing the lesion itself as well as bronchial, hilar, and mediastinal involvement.[20]

The advent of computed tomography (CT) and its ability to distinguish small differences in radiation attenuation in tissue has led to the thought that CT may be applied in the differentiation of benign and malignant pulmonary disease. The initial experience of Siegelman et al. with 91 lung nodules has shown that lesions with CT numbers over 164 H(Hounsfield) are benign.[21] Since both malignant and benign pulmonary lesions may contain calcium,[22] additional studies are needed to corroborate this diagnostic technique. Furthermore, reports indicate that CT can be of benefit in detecting multiplicity of lesions, subpleural metastatic disease, pleural versus extrapleural lesions, the vascular nature of lesions by utilizing contrast enhancement, etc.[23,24]

Of special significance is the major benefit of CT in evaluation of the mediastinum. Anterior tracheal, subcarinal, and cardiophrenic angle nodes are well visualized. The hilar areas are viewed so that adenopathy can be detected whether it extends laterally, anteriorly, or posteriorly. Recently, the usefulness of CT regarding the diagnosis of inflammatory and neoplastic diseases arising from or affecting the bronchi has been emphasized.[25] The CT number of mediastinal lesions can be extremely helpful in excluding surgery for fatty masses or diffuse mediastinal widening secondary to fatty deposition.[26]

In spite of the above, there still is not a concensus opinion as to whether conventional or computed tomography should be performed in any given instance to obtain the most beneficial information.

The distinction of benign and malignant may be further aided by fiberoptic bronchoscopy.[27,28] Accuracy rates have been reported in the 70 to 80 percent range. Percutaneous lung biopsy has also been popularized, with the procedure being relatively easily accomplished, especially with the use of the "skinny needle."[29,30] Of major importance is the fact that specimens from these various biopsy techniques can save unnecessary treatment, surgery, or further work-up. In order to do so, however, people must be available who are experienced in cytologic preparation and interpretation of these small specimens.

In general, ultrasound is not as useful in the chest as in the abdomen, due to the dampening effect of sound transmission through aerated lung. Nevertheless, ultrasound may be useful in the differentiation (and localization) of pleural thickening and fluid. Another application might conceivably be derived from the scanning of mediastinal lesions via a probe within the esophagus. Ultrasound can prove useful over and above CT in distinguishing solid from cystic mediastinal or chest wall lesions when CT numbers do not provide definitive information.

Staging

Within the last few years, staging of lung carcinoma to determine surgical resectability has received much attention.[31,32] In this respect, radiologic imaging can be of tremendous importance, since even with cervical mediastinoscopy, the hilar and subcarinal areas are not as easily accessible as the paratracheal and subcervical nodes. In addition, since the aortic–pulmonic window area must be approached by a parasternal incision, radiologic evaluation of this area prior to surgery is essential.

Full lung tomography is an excellent method for evaluating the extent of disease, since additional parenchymal involvement may be found as well as mediastinal spread. CT offers an even further opportunity to evaluate subcarinal, anterior tracheal, and cardiophrenic angle nodes and for clarifying questionable areas on routine tomography.

As concerns the lung parenchyma, CT can demonstrate additional nodules and be of help in determining the extent of a tumor. In one study of 29 patients studied with whole lung tomography, CT scans of 10 patients detected additional nodules.[23] In another report, 5 of 60 patients with a history of malignant tumor demonstrated nodules on CT that were undetected on plain radiographs or conventional tomograms.[24] Unfortunately, in many areas of the country, these additional nodules turn out to be small granulomatous lesions and therefore an inappropriate diagnosis of unresectability could result. Subpleural metastatic disease, however, is best evaluated by CT. The potential for all radiologic imaging techniques in the staging evaluation of the T (tumor), N (nodal), and M (metastatic) categories of lung cancer is great. Future efforts need to be directed toward refinements in making these staging efforts more accurate and specific.

RECOMMENDATIONS FOR RESEARCH SUPPORT

Viewer Perception.   Viewer perception has received attention in the literature, but many unanswered questions remain.[33] Potentially fruitful areas for investigation would include evaluation of optimal light intensities, viewer techniques, distraction or distractors on film, concepts of structured noise, and lesion conspicuity. The psychophysical aspects of human vision, such as retinal brightness and contrast adaptation, also offer potential areas of investigation. Such knowledge would be extremely useful in improvement of present modalities and in the design of newer radiographic techniques.

Priority: 1
Duration: 1 to 5 years
Probability of Success: high

Improving Techniques in Chest Radiography.   In spite of extensive work on chest radiographic techniques,[6,34,35] no "optimal" technique exists. Further work could prove rewarding, including:

1. Investigation of film–screen combinations to optimize nodule detection at low radiation doses.
2. Highly efficient scatter rejection techniques to improve radiographic contrast, such as moving slit radiography and improved grids.[36]
3. Image modification, such as unsharp masking,[37] to improve image contrast.

4. Computer techniques, including image or display modification[38] and computed radiography.

Priority: 1
Duration: ongoing
Probability of Success: high

Biopsy Techniques.   Multi-institutional trials are needed both to compare existing fiberoptic and "skinny needle" biopsy techniques and to train personnel in the performance of these procedures. Investigations into other possible methods or refinements of existing techniques in sampling lung tissue could conceivably result in improved accuracy in the diagnosis of malignant disease at an earlier stage. Finally, improved specificity must result from existing staging procedures.

Priority: 1
Duration: ongoing
Probability of Success: high

Comparison of Present Modalities.   A multi-institutional study comparing conventional kVp technique, 350 kVp technique, conventional tomography, and CT should be implemented with regard to accuracy of nodule detection. In addition, comparison should be made as to the ability of these techniques to determine whether the nodule is benign or malignant and the accuracy of staging. Further investigation into the possibility of reducing mottle and focal spot size with 350 kVp technique would also be helpful.

Priority: 1
Duration: 2 to 3 years
Probability of Success: high

CT in Lung Nodule Diagnosis.   Siegelman et al. recently reported their experience with CT in the evaluation of 88 patients with 91 nodular pulmonary lesions. Representative CT numbers of 164 H or greater occurred only with benign lesions. CT numbers of 147 H or below are within the range of malignancy.[21]

A multi-institutional trial is needed to further evaluate this diagnostic technique, using different CT units, a broader and larger sample of solitary pulmonary nodules, and different patient and physician settings.

Priority: 1
Duration: 2 to 3 years
Probability of Success: high

Positive Sputum Cytology and Normal Chest X-ray: T_x Lung Cancer Patient. The institutional trial programs currently under way have domonstrated the frequency of occurrence of the sputum cytology positive–x-ray negative patient (T_x stage lung cancer). Additional efforts are necessary to improve our ability to localize these occult tumors prior to their appearance on the chest x-ray. Multi-institutional studies comparing magnification radiography, subtraction techniques, computer enhancement, selective bronchography, and bronchoscopy are needed.

Priority: 1
Duration: 3 years
Probability of Success: moderate

Tumor Labeling. The prospects of immunologic application to the identification and determination of the extent of pulmonary malignancy may offer new avenues of investigation. Labeling of tumors with agents may offer more definitive evidence of benignity versus malignancy and might be applicable not only to CT but also to nuclear radiologic imaging of the chest.[39]

Priority: 2
Duration: 5 years
Probability of Success: moderate

ACKNOWLEDGMENT

Gratitude is expressed to Dr. Richard Greenspan, Department of Diagnostic Radiology, Yale University Medical School, for reveiw of this chapter.

REFERENCES

1. Seidman H, Silverberg E, Holleb AI: Cancer statistics, 1976: A comparison of white and black populations. Cancer 26:2–30, 1976.

2. Benfield JR, Juillard GJF, Pilch YH, et al: Current and future concepts of lung cancer. Ann Intern Med 83:93–106, 1975.
3. Sagel SS, Evens RG, Forrest JV, Bramson RD: Accuracy of routine screening and lateral chest radiographs in a hospital-based population. N Engl J Med 291:1001–1004, 1974.
4. Garland LH: The rate of growth and natural duration of primary bronchial cancer. Am J Roentgenol 96:604–611, 1966.
5. Thomas RG, Wiles SJ, Sluis-Cremer GK: Chest radiography at 200 kV. S Afr Med J 48:2465–2568, 1974.
6. Proto AV, Lane EJ: 350 kVp chest radiography: Review and comparison with 120 kVp. Am J Roentgenol 130:859–866, May 1978.
7. Judkins MP, Abrams HL, Bristow JD, et al: Report of the Intersociety Commission for Heart Disease Resources: Optimal resources for examination of the chest and cardiovascular system. Circulation 53:A1–A37, 1976.
8. Ting YM, Doust BD, Chuang VP: Xerotomographic diagnosis of central bronchogenic carcinoma. Chest 67:172–175, 1975.
9. Harle TS, Hevezi JM, Rogers LF, et al: Xerotomography of the tracheobronchial tree. Am J Roentgenol 124:353–357, 1975.
10. Lefcoe MS: Direct magnification in radiography of the chest in diffuse pulmonary disease. J Can Assoc Radiol 27:3–8, 1976.
11. Christensen E: An Introduction to the Physics of Diagnostic Radiology, ed 2. Lea & Febiger, 1978, p 294.
12. Milne ENC: The role and performance of minute focal spots in roentgenology with special reference to magnification. Crit Rev Radiol Sci 2:269–280, 1971.
13. Fontana RS, Sanderson DR, Woolner LB, et al: Mayo lung project for early detection and localization of bronchogenic carcinoma: A status report. Chest 67:511–522, 1975.
14. Melamed M, Flehinger B, Miller D, et al: Preliminary report of lung cancer detection program in New York. Cancer 39:369–382, 1977.
15. Schlesinger RB, Schweizer RD, Cahng TL, et al: Controlled deposition of tantalum powder in a case of the human airways: Applications for aerosol bronchography. Invest Radiol 10:115–123, May–April 1975.
16. Hinchcliffe WA, Zamel N, Fishman NH, et al: Roentgenographic study of the human trachea with powdered tantalum. Radiology 97:327–330, 1970.
17. Charles Putman: Personal communication, 1979.
18. Hessel SJ, Herman PG, Swensson RG: Improving performance by multiple interpretations of chest radiographs: Effectiveness and cost. Radiology 127:589–594, 1978.
19. Littleton J: Tomography: Physical Principals and Clinical Applications. Baltimore, Williams and Wilkins, 1976.
20. Brown LR, DeRemee RA: 55° Oblique hilar tomography. Mayo Clin Proc 51:89–95, 1976.
21. Siegelman SS, Zerhouni EA, Leo FP, et al: CT of the solitary pulmonary nodule. Am J Roentgenol 135:1–13, July 1980.
22. Proto AV: Radiology of the chest, in Wilson GH (ed): Current Radiology. Boston, Houghton Mifflin Professional Publishers, 1978, vol 1.
23. Muhn JR, Brown LR, Crowe JK: Detection of pulmonary nodules by computed tomography. Am J Roentgenol 128:267–270, 1977.
24. Jost RG, Sagel SS, Stanley RJ, Levitt RG: Computed tomography of the thorax. Radiology 126:125–136, 1978.

25. Naidich DP, Stitik FP, Khouri NF, et al: Computed tomography of the bronchi:II. Pathology. J Comp Assist Tomogr 4:754–762, 1980.
26. Heitzman ER, Goldwin RL, Proto AV: Radiologic analysis of the mediastinum utilizing computed tomography. Radiol Clin North Am 15:309–329, 1977.
27. Kvale PA, Bode FR, Kini S: Diagnostic accuracy in lung cancer: Comparison of techniques used in association with flexible fiberoptic bronchoscopy. Chest 69:732–736, 1976.
28. Marsh BR, Frost JQ, Erozan YS, et al: Flexible fiberoptic bronchoscopy: Its place in the search for lung cancer. Ann Otol 82:757–764, 1973.
29. Herman PG, Hessel SJ: The diagnostic accuracy and complication of closed lung biopsies. Radiology 125:11–14, 1977.
30. Nick R, Heard BE, Hinson KF, et al: Aspiration needle biopsy of thoracic lesions: An assessment of 227 biopsies. Br J Dis Chest 68:86–94, 1974.
31. Carr DT, Mountain CF: The staging of lung cancer. Semin Oncol 1:229–234, 1974.
32. Mountain CF, Carr DT, Anderson WAD: Clinical staging of lung cancer. Am J Roentgenol 120:130–138, 1974.
33. Kundel HL: Radiological image perception. Appl Radiol March–April 1975, pp 27–31.
34. Jacobson G, Bohlig H, Kiviluoto R: Essentials of chest radiography. Radiology 95:445–450, 1970.
35. Wilkinson GA, Fraser RG: Roentgenography of the chest. Appl Radiol May/June 1976, pp 41–49.
36. Sorenson JA, Nelson JA: Investigations of moving-slit radiography. Radiology 120:705–711, 1976.
37. Nelson JA, Niklason L, Sorenson JA: Application of lung masking technique to chest radiography. Invest Radiol 14:380, 1979.
38. Idstrom LG, Bower EH: The digital computer in diagnostic radiology. Appl Radiol 7:51–56, July–August 1978.
39. Kono M, Yoshida Y, Sako M, et al: Tomography and hilar lymphadenography: Significance in the diagnosis of lung cancer and its extent. Nippon Acta Radiol 37:665–676, 1977.

EIGHT

Gastrointestinal Tumors

Gerald D. Dodd
and
Bernard E. Zeligman

INTRODUCTION AND BACKGROUND

Until recently, the role of the diagnostic radiologist in digestive tract neoplasia has largely been confined to the demonstration of symptomatic disease. The futility of this approach is indicated by the survival rates obtained in most sites.[1] The observed 5 year survival rates (male and female) for all ages and stages of disease are as follows:

Esophagus	3%
Stomach	9%
Pancreas	1%
Liver	2%
Gallbladder and ducts	6%

Less than 50 percent of the tumors in the above categories are resectable. It is not until the colon and rectum are considered that appreciable results are apparent. The overall 5 year survival rate for patients under 45 years of age is 59 percent. This decreases to 20 percent for those 75 years of age and older. However, over 70 percent of all colon cancers diagnosed may be classified as localized or regional disease. This is reflected in the low percentage of unresectable cases (17 percent) and an overall 5 year survival rate of 50 percent. The differences in the survival rates with disease of the colorectum and disease in other portions of the gastrointestinal tract must reflect fundamental differences in the biologic potential of the individual tumors. Nevertheless, it would appear that improved

81

survival rates may be anticipated in other portions of the gut as the percentage of localized disease diagnosed increases.[2]

Current radiologic techniques are capable of detecting gastrointestinal neoplasms that are limited to the mucosa and submucosa. While these techniques are susceptible to improvement, the major problem is the lack of guidelines by which to apply them. Carcinoma of the esophagus, for example, represents only 7 percent of all gastrointestinal cancers, and in recent years the incidence of carcinoma of the stomach has declined to 9 per 100,000, approximately 1/30 that of breast cancer. These low incidences, coupled with the costs of the examinations and the potential dangers of radiation, sharply limit the use of standard radiologic methods for screening and early detection. Obviously, the efficacy of the techniques could be improved by better definition of the suspect populations.

Since carcinoma of the colorectum constitutes about 55 percent of all gastrointestinal cancers, the yield for screening procedures in this area is higher. In addition, certain markers—such as familial history, increased CEA titers, and/or a positive hematest—further increase the case-finding capabilities of the radiographic examination. The double contrast enema probably represents the most successful application of diagnostic radiologic techniques to the early detection of gastrointestinal cancers; it has the potential of identifying the majority of tumors prior to their spread beyond the colonic wall. The patient survival rates for such tumors are very high and should equal those achieved by the Japanese with superficial gastroneoplasms—i.e., 90 to 95 percent.[2]

STATE OF THE ART

Gut

Esophagus. The development of double contrast esophagography has made possible the detection of small mucosal abnormalities.[3-6] Unfortunately, the esophagus does not have a serosa and therefore involvement of the mediastinal structures may occur early in the development of a tumor. There are presently few data as to the influence of treatment upon these morphologically limited lesions, but the anatomic peculiarities of the esophagus may well limit the impact of early detection in this area.[7]

Stomach. Under optimum conditions, double contrast examination of the stomach and duodenum is a sensitive tool.[8-14] As demonstrated by the Japanese, it is possible to discover extremely small and superficial cancers with an ensuing 90 to 95 percent 5 year survival rate.[2] Glucagon and Pro-Banthīne are effective in producing transient gastric paralysis, which, when coupled with the distention of the organ by ingested gas, obliterates the major mucosal pattern and permits minute evaluation of the mucosal surface. The minor mucosal pattern (area gastricae) is demonstrable in approximately 50 percent of patients, allowing an even more precise estimate of the integrity of the mucous membrane. With proper film coverage, all portions of the stomach and duodenum may be visualized, and because of the inhibition of motion, fluoroscopic evaluation of motility is neither possible nor necessary. Fluoroscopy is therefore used only for positioning the patient, a factor which substantially decreases dose. The capabilities of the technique have been well demonstrated by Laufer, who has shown an excellent correlation between endoscopy and the double contrast barium meal.[15] This correlation has extended to lesions as small as 2 to 3 mm in diameter.

Computed tomography (CT) and ultrasound have also demonstrated gastric tumors. These modalities have demonstrated large primary gastric cancers and some metastases and may therefore come to have some value in assessing extragastric extent. However, these modalities have not demonstrated small primary cancers.[16]

Small Intestine. Neoplasia of the small intestine is uncommon, and, while modern barium preparations allow a reasonably thorough examination of the small bowel, the infrequency of tumors makes it the least productive in terms of yield. Nevertheless, the recently revived small bowel enema has made earlier and more precise diagnoses of all diseases possible.[17-20]

Colon. Double contrast examination of the colon has been developed to a fine art, predominantly through the efforts of Welin and Welin and Miller.[21,22] While modern barium preparations have had a pronounced effect upon the quality of the examination, the basic improvements have resulted from adequate attention to preparation of the bowel, realization of the necessity for multiprojectional coverage, and the adoption of double contrast technique.

With a properly performed double contrast enema, 3 to 5 mm polyps can be detected. Indeed, approximately 90 percent of polyps detected by colonoscopy can be demonstrated by double contrast technique. Furthermore, some polyps undetected by colonoscopy can be demonstrated by the enema.[23-25] The high rate of demonstration of polypoid lesions is important for diagnosing not only early cancers but also the adenomatous polyp, a lesion which may well be the precursor of most colonic cancers.[26,27]

Some value of CT for colonic carcinoma imaging has been demonstrated. A limitation of the barium enema is its failure to demonstrate in the pelvis or abdomen some recurrences of colonic malignancy. CT can detect some of these recurrences.[28]

Liver and Pancreas

CT and ultrasound have advanced significantly the imaging of liver and pancreatic neoplasms. Comparisons of scintigraphy, ultrasonography, and CT in patients with liver disease indicates that CT is the most accurate of the three modalities in the identification of mass and the assessment of the extent of hepatic disease. When used in combination, CT and scintigraphy are most effective; gas or excessive fat may interfere with the formation of an adequate ultrasonic image. The sensitivity of arteriography for smaller tumors exceeds that of the other procedures, but only if the tumors are vascular. In the presence of avascular disease, the noninvasive techniques are superior. For practical purposes, all of these methods are complementary, but in daily use arteriography is reserved for those cases in which definitive information is required and the other imaging techniques have yielded negative results.[29,30] Unfortunately, the newer diagnostic methods have not significantly increased the number of early diagnoses, and most malignant liver tumors are metastatic. Therefore, these methods have not affected mortality rates. They are primarily of value in determining the stage of the disease.

Until recently, detection of pancreatic tumors has depended largely upon their effect on adjacent structures or on the arteriographic demonstration of vessel encasement, vessel displacement, tumor stain, etc. In the main, these techniques are useful only with advanced tumors and have done little to increase survival rates. Scintigraphy has also been unsatisfactory because of poor imaging characteristics of the available radiopharmaceutical and nonspecificity of a positive scan.

The recent introduction of ultrasound and computed tomography scanning has modified this picture somewhat. Smaller primary neoplasms are identifiable in all parts of the pancreas as a result of changes in outline or bulk of the organ. Because it depicts the entirety of the gland more often, CT has somewhat more successfully demonstrated pancreatic tumors. CT also better demonstrates retropancreatic spread of tumor. Despite these advances, however, major problems of specificity and sensitivity remain.[31-33]

Endoscopic retrograde cholangiopancreatography (ERCP) is the only method of demonstrating in detail the pancreatic ducts and is highly accurate.[34] Rarely is the ERCP negative when a tumor is present. A specific diagnosis of cancer cannot always be made, however, and the procedure is cumbersome.[35,36]

Percutaneous aspiration biopsy is becoming closely allied to pancreatic and liver tumor imaging. This biopsy technique has increased the specificity of imaging methods and, in turn, is more helpful when guided by an image. Safe percutaneous biopsy has become feasible since the introduction of the Chiba needle. While various imaging modalities have been used successfully in directing the needle to the lesion, [37-39] ultrasound [40] and CT [41] have been particularly helpful, with CT the more helpful of the two. This image-directed biopsy technique is reducing significantly the number of more invasive procedures for diagnosing tumors of these organs.

LIMITATIONS OF CURRENT TECHNIQUES AND EQUIPMENT

Roentgenographic Examinations
The majority of radiologic procedures involving the gastrointestinal tract utilize both fluoroscopy and radiography. The combination of the two techniques yields exposures considerably in excess of most standard radiographic procedures. Tradition more or less requires fluoroscopic evaluation of the section of the gastrointestinal tract in question, followed by films which are frequently made by technicians. These technician-directed exams are often inadequate or noninformative. While this sequence was defensible prior to the introduction of the image intensifier and modern spot-filming techniques, there are currently no data which clearly support or refute this approach.

Gut

Esophagus. Although contrast material is easily introduced into the esophagus, the examination is frequently difficult due to the rapid passage of the opaque material. It has been suggested that double contrast techniques are superior to conventional single contrast studies, but the shortcomings of the various procedures may be summarized as follows:

1. Lack of an adequate esophageal paralytic agent.
2. The transient nature of the coating of the esophagus by contrast agents, particularly when double contrast techniques are employed.
3. Inadequate means of introducing air into the esophagus for double contrast examination.
4. Lack of information concerning the reproducibility of double contrast techniques.
5. Lack of statistical proof of the increased effectiveness of double contrast examination as compared with conventional radiographic and fluoroscopic techniques.

Stomach. Although the double contrast examination is reputed to significantly increase the sensitivity of the upper gastrointestinal examination,
there are many unresolved problems:

1. The control of gastric secretion.
2. Incompatibility of gastric secretions with available contrast media.
3. Unequal coating of the mucous membrane due to the physical
   properties of the contrast media.
4. Crude methods of air induction for double contrast techniques.
5. Lack of clinical experimental data which document the reputed
   advantage of double contrast gastrography over conventional single
   contrast techniques.
6. Lack of documented information concerning the number and types
   of films required to assure adequate coverage of the stomach.
7. Lack of statistical proof of the adequacy or inadequacy of double
   contrast techniques in the examination of the duodenum.

Small Intestine. The use of modern barium preparations has largely
obviated problems related to precipitation of barium within the small
intestine. However, there are still difficulties in this respect during pro-
tracted examinations, and the newer contrast media have not affected the
problem of superimposition of intestinal loops. While the latter may be
minimized by the small intestinal enema, intubation of the stomach and
duodenum is time-consuming, expensive, and unpleasant for the patient.
Fortunately, the incidence of small bowel neoplasia is so low that this
does not constitute a significant problem in detection.

Colon. The double contrast enema is an extremely sensitive examination, the utility of which is limited by the lack of appreciation on the part
of physicians for the need for absolute cleansing of the bowel. Related
problems include:

1. Inadequate comparison of individual cleansing regimes. There is no
   reliable statistical information as to the relative capability of one or
   more cleansing protocols.
2. Variability in the physical properties of the barium sulfate suspensions.
3. Paralytic agents available for barium enema examinations are mar-
   ginal in effect and often fail to control an irritable bowel.
4. Patient discomfort.

Liver, Spleen, and Pancreas
Tumors less than 2 cm in diameter are usually not detectable by nuclear
scanning. Ultrasound and CT have theoretically greater levels of resolu-

tion, but are section dependent—i.e., chance plays a role in the detection of tumors under 1 cm in diameter, since the smaller neoplasms may lie between the planes of the individual scans. While those tumors large enough to alter the size and contour of the gland are readily detected by these techniques, they are frequently far advanced. There is also no precise specificity for tissue type, a fact which limits the capability of these techniques.

The need exists for discovery of pancreatic neoplasm before it enlarges or deforms the normal outline of the gland. An imaging agent whose target organ is primarily the pancreas is needed in order to delineate smaller mass lesions. The advent of CT, with its ability to demonstrate minute differences in radiographic densities, suggests that binding of a high atomic number atom to such agents as amino acids or others specific for the pancreas could produce earlier diagnosis.

Although arteriography is an inherently hazardous procedure, it has a greater degree of sensitivity than ultrasound and CT for vascular tumors. At the present time, there are no reliable data as to the comparative efficacy of these techniques in the small, avascular neoplasm. Unquestionably, the best results may be obtained by a combination of the three, but the cost is difficult to justify.

Biliary Tract

Oral and intravenous contrast media are useful in the diagnosis of biliary tract calculi but are of limited value in neoplastic disease. Percutaneous cholangiography affords precise information but is potentially hazardous and requires hospitalization.[42-45] Endoscopic retrograde cholangiopancreatography (ERCP) provides another method of visualization of the biliary tract, but in view of the success obtained with percutaneous cholangiography, ERCP for visualization of the biliary tract is becoming less important.[46]

Recently, CT and ultrasound have permitted diagnosis of carcinoma of the gallbladder. This neoplasm has been difficult to diagnose with other modalities, often presenting as nonopacification of the gallbladder or oral cholecystogram, and the diagnosis has therefore often been made at surgery when cholecystitis was suspected. However, most of these tumors diagnosed with CT or ultrasound have been advanced tumors. No impact on survival has been demonstrated.[47-50]

Intravenous and oral contrast media have little application in the diagnosis of tumors of the biliary tract. Jaundice is often the presenting symptom, and these contrast agents are largely ineffective in the presence of clinical icterus. Percutaneous cholangiography with 17 to 20 gauge needles is hazardous due to such complications as hemorrhage, systemic sepsis, and bile peritonitis. The introduction of the Chiba needle has reduced this risk and made routine use of the procedure feasible. Nevertheless, complications do occur, and hospitalization is required for the examination.

Endoscopic retrograde cholangiopancreatography is cumbersome and is of primary usefulness in visualization of the pancreatic duct. ERCP may be attempted if percutaneous cholangiography is unsuccessful.

RECOMMENDATIONS FOR RESEARCH SUPPORT

Equipment
Potential solutions to the problem of patient dose include:

1. Omission of fluoroscopy except for purposes of positioning the patient.
2. Omission of conventional radiography with the substitution of direct photography or videotape recording of the output phosphor of the image intensifier.
3. The replacement of conventional screen–film combinations by rare-earth screens and high speed film.

With the above in mind, the following areas of research are recommended:

1. Improvement of image intensifier systems with the goals of maintenance of image quality and concomitant dose reduction per unit of time.
2. The improvement of output phosphor photographic and taping techniques, from the standpoints of both image quality and the size of the recorded image.
3. The investigation of various screen–film combinations in an attempt to further minimize dose while maintaining the necessary degree of resolution and detail.

All of the above require the cooperation of industry. While advances of this type are a natural activity of private industry, the problem of dose is so important that the active participation of a federal agency would do much to speed their availability. These projects should have a high priority and the probability of success are excellent. Approximately 3 to 5 years would be needed for completion.

Priority: 1
Duration: 3 to 5 years
Probability of Success: excellent

Another area for research would involve prospective randomized studies comparing the efficacy of combined fluoroscopy and radiography, as opposed to the use of film or videotape alone. Filming techniques should include direct photography of the output phosphor of the image intensifier. Colonoscopy and gastroscopy should be used as controls in an effort to determine the most efficacious method of examination at the least risk and expense to the patient.

These considerations are relevant and should have a reasonably high priority. The materials are at hand and clinical trials at institutions performing large numbers of gastrointestinal examinations should be easily initiated. Substantive information should be derived in two to three years, and the probabilities of significant benefits in terms of reduced population dose, diagnostic efficacy, and cost control are high.

Priority: 1
Duration: 2 to 3 years
Probability of Success: high

Methods of Examination

There is no clear-cut evidence of the superiority of double contrast techniques over the more conventional single contrast method. Large-scale double blind studies directed toward establishing the relative efficacy of these two techniques in the various portions of the gastrointestinal tract would be of importance. Any such investigations should include the following elements.

Contrast Media. The development of new contrast materials is a complex procedure. Despite many attempts since the turn of the century, barium has not been replaced as the basic agent. Although the benefits which might be gained from a new medium are potentially great, it is estimated that at least 5 to 10 years of effort would be required to produce a useful compound, with the probabilities of success only moderate.

The properties of barium sulfate and its proper use have been incompletely explored. Barium sulfate preparations vary in particle size, tendency to clump, viscosity, etc. Documentation of optimum particle size, viscosity, concentration, etc. for a specific type of examination should be of great value and allow the potential of the contrast medium to be completely developed.

Barium suspensions are also frequently modified by the gastrointestinal contents. The development of pharmacologic agents which would limit or suspend secretory functions or agents with mucolytic properties would be of considerable use in assuring the efficacy of an examination.

Gas-producing Agents. The development of gas-producing agents which may be easily ingested, produce large quantities of gas, and minimize bubble formation should have priority. Extension of the work of James et al. concerning the methods of introducing gas into the stomach would be useful.[10] In their series of patients, five methods were used and effervescent tablets seemed to have a clear statistical edge over the others.

Antifoam Agents. Antifoam agents are indispensible in minimizing or eliminating bubble formation in the double contrast examination. There is, however, no precise information concerning the optimum quantity to use for a specific type of examination. Unquestionably, excessive amounts can interfere with the coating properties of the contrast medium, and too little is ineffective in preventing bubble formation. There is a similar lack of information concerning the interaction of simethicone and related agents with the various barium sulfate preparations. This type of information is essential to the performance of acceptable contrast procedures.

Filming Techniques. There are no controlled studies which indicate the number and type of films necessary to assure an adequate examination of a specific portion of the gastrointestinal tract. This is true of both the single and double contrast techniques. Structured studies which would permit a precise evaluation of the individual projections and their contribution to the total examination would be of value from the standpoints of diagnostic accuracy, patient dose, and cost.

Radiographic Magnification. Magnification techniques for the examination of the mucosa of the gastrointestinal tract should be investigated as an aid to the early detection and identification of neoplasms. Pertinent examples include interruption of the pattern of the area gastrica in the stomach as an indication of the early mucosal destruction and the demonstration of dysplasia in the colon as a precursor of carcinoma in chronic ulcerative colitis.[51]

Present x-ray tubes for magnification radiography are unable to sustain the high potentials required for ultrashort exposures. The development of microfocus tubes capable of operating at higher energies should have moderately high priority. The eventual success of any such program is directly related to the efficacy of the contrast medium and therefore should proceed in parallel with developments in contrast media.

All of the foregoing considerations are highly relevant and are directly applicable to the accuracy and safety of a given gastrointestinal examination. Such programs would require 2 to 4 years of structure and produce suitable numbers of examinations. The probability of obtaining useful information is excellent.

Priority: 1
Duration: 2 to 4 years
Probability of Success: excellent

Nonimaging Methods

Current imaging techniques are not suitable for screening the entire population for early, asymptomatic gastrointestinal cancer. Therefore, in addition to further investigations for improving imaging techniques, investigation into means of selecting for imaging those people most likely to harbor a gastrointestinal malignancy should be a high priority.

This approach would be valuable for all organs of the gastrointestinal tract. However, because diagnosis of early colorectal carcinoma has been shown to significantly improve survival rates, and because the double contrast enema can detect early cancer, this tumor should receive the highest priority. Furthermore, the adenomatous polyp, accepted by many as the precursor of most colonic carcinomas, can usually be detected with the double contrast enema. Studies of various screening methods are currently under way. Preliminary results suggest that testing people over 50 years of age for occult focal blood may in part select the appropriate population for further evaluation, including a double contrast enema, to detect early, asymptomatic malignancies or premalignant lesions of the colon.[52]

Priority: 1
Duration: ongoing, but to assess the effect of polyp removal
on the death rate from colonic carcinoma could require 10
years or more.

ACKNOWLEDGMENT

Gratitude is expressed to Dr. Jeff O. Janes, Department of Radiology, University of Utah College of Medicine, for review of this chapter.

REFERENCES

 1. Axtell LM, Cutler SJ, Myers MH (eds): End Results in Cancer. Report No. 4, Prepared by End Results Section, Biometry Branch, National Cancer Institute, US Department of HEW, Bethesda, Md, DHEW Publication (NIH) 73-272.
 2. Kidokoro T: Frequently of resection, metastasis and five-year survival rate of early gastric carcinoma in a surgical clinic, in Murakami T (ed): Early Gastric Cancer. Japanese Cancer Association, GANN Monograph on Cancer Research No. 11, pp 45–49, Tokyo, 1972.
 3. Goldstein H, Dodd GD: Double contrast examination of the esophagus. Gastrointest Radiol 1:3–6, 1976.
 4. Itai Y, Kogure T, Okuyama Y: Superficial esophageal carcinoma. Radiology 6:597–691, 1978.
 5. Koehler RE, Moss AA, Margulis AR: Early radiographic manifestations of carcinoma of the esophagus. Radiology 119:1–5, 1976.
 6. Yamada A: Radiologic assessment of resectability and prognosis in esophageal carcinoma. Gastrointest Radiol 4:213–218, 1979.
 7. Zornoza J, Lindell MM Jr.: Radiologic evaluation of small esophageal carcinoma. Gastrointest Radiol 5:107–111, 1980.
 8. Gelfand DW, Hachiya J: The double contrast examination of the stomach using gas-producing granules and tablets. Radiology 98:1381–1382, 1969.
 9. Goldstein H: Double contrast gastrography. Am J Dig Dis 29:797–803, 1976.
10. James WB, McCreath G, Sutherland GR, et al: Double contrast barium meal examination. Clin Radiol 27:99–101, 1976.
11. Kreel L, Herlinger H, Glanville J: Techniques of the double contrast barium meal with examples of correlations with endoscopy. Clin Radiol ?⁴·307–314, 1973.
12. Laufer I: A simple method for routine double contrast study of the upper gastrointestinal tract. Radiology 117:513–518, 1975.
13. Obata WG: A double contrast technique for examination of the stomach using gas-producing granules and tablets. Radiology 93:1381–1382, 1969.
14. Shirakabe H, et al: Atlas of X-ray Diagnosis of Early Gastric Cancer. Philadelphia, Lippincott, 1966.
15. Laufer I: Assessment of the accuracy of double contrast gastroduodenal radiology. Gastroenterology 71:874–878, 1976.
16. Komaiko MS: Gastric neoplasm: Ultrasound and CT evaluation. Gastrointest Radiol 4:131–137, 1979.
17. Miller RE, Sellink JL: Enteroclysis: The small bowel enema—how to succeed, how to fail. Exhibit at RSNA, 1977.
18. Novak D: Double-contrast examination of the small bowel without intubation. Fortschr Geb Roentgenstr Nuklearmed 125:38–41, 1976.
19. Saunders DE, Ho CS: The small bowel enema: Experience with 150 examinations. Am J Roentgenol 127:743–751, 1976.
20. Sellink JL: Radiologic examination of the small intestine by duodenal intubation. Acta Radiol (Diagn) 15:318–331, 1974.
21. Welin S, Welin G: The Double Contrast Examination of the Colon: Experiences with the Welin Modification. Stuttgart, Germany, Georg Thieme Verlag, 1976.
22. Miller RE: Examination of the Colon. Curr Probl Radiol 5 (2):3–4, 1975.

23. Laufer I, Smith NCW, Mullens JE: The radiological demonstration of colorectal polyps undetected by endoscopy. Gastroenterology 70:167–170, 1976.
24. Ott DJ, Gelfand DW, Wu WC, et al: Sensitivity of double-contrast barium enema: Emphasis on polyp detection. Am J Roentgenol 135:327–330, 1980.
25. Theoni RF, Menuck L: Comparison of barium enema and colonoscopy in the detection of small colonic polyps. Radiology 124:631–634, 1977.
26. Lane N, Fenoglio CM: The adenoma–carcinoma sequence in the stomach and colon: 1. Observations on the adenoma as precursor to ordinary large bowel carcinoma. Gastrointest Radiol 1:111–119, 1976.
27. Morson B: The polyp–cancer sequence in the large bowel. Proc R Soc Med 67:451–457, 1974.
28. Husband JE, Hodson NJ, Parsons CA: The use of computed tomography in recurrent rectal tumors. Radiology 134:677–682, 1980.
29. Snow JH, Goldstein HM, Wallace S: Comparison of scintigraphy, ultrasonography and computed tomography in the evaluation of hepatic neoplasms. Am J Roentgenol 132:915–918, 1979.
30. MacCarty RL, Stephens DH, Hattery RR, et al: Hepatic imaging by computed tomography: A comparison with ^{99m} Tc-sulfur colloid, ultrasonography, and angiography. Radiol Clin North Am 17:137–155, 1979.
31. Foley WD, Stewart ET, Lawson TL, et al: Computed tomography, ultrasonography, and endoscopic retrograde cholangiopancreatography in the diagnosis of pancreatic disease: A comparative study. Gastrointest Radiol 5:29–35. 1980.
32. Lee JKT, Stanley RJ, Melson GL, et al: Pancreatic imaging by ultrasound and computed tomography: A general review. Radiol Clin North Am 17:105–117, 1979.
33. Whalen JP: Radiology of the abdomen: Impact of new imaging methods. Am J Roentgenol 133:585–618, 1979.
34. Freeny PC, Bilbao MK, Katon RM: "Blind" evaluation of endoscopic retrograde cholangiography (ERCP) in the diagnosis of pancreatic carcinoma: The "double duct" and other signs. Diag Radiol 119:271–274, 1976.
35. Gregg, JA, Gramm HF, Clouse ME: Problems in the diagnosis of pancreatic carcinoma by endoscopic retrograde cholangiopancreatography. Gastrointest Radiol 2:61–65, 1977.
36. Ralls PW, Halls, IJ, Renner I: Endoscopic retrograde cholangiopancreatography (ERCP) in pancreatic disease. Radiology 134:347–352, 1980.
37. Goldstein HM, Zornoza, J, Wallace S, et al: Percutaneous fine needle aspiration biopsy of pancreatic and other abdominal masses. Radiology 123:319–322, 1977.
38. Tylen U, Arnesjo B, Lindberg LG, et al: Percutaneous biopsy of carcinoma of the pancreas guided by angiography. Surg Gynecol Obstet 142:737–739, 1976.
39. Zornoza J, Wallace S, Ordonez N, et al: Fine-needle aspiration biopsy of the liver. Am J Roentgenol 134:331–334, 1980.
40. Skolnick ML, Dekker A, Weinstein BJ: Ultrasound guided fine-needle aspiration biopsy of abdominal masses. Gastrointest Radiol 3:295–302, 1978.
41. Ferrucci JT Jr, Wittenberg J: CT biopsy of abdominal tumors: Aids for lesion localization. Radiology 129:739–744, 1978.
42. Burcharth F, Christiansen L, Efsen F, et al: Percutaneous transhepatic cholangiography in diagnostic evaluation of 160 jaundiced patients. Am J Surg 133:559–561, 1977.

43. Ferrucci JT, Wittenberg J, Sarno RA, et al: Fine needle transhepatic cholangiography: A new approach to obstructive jaundice. Am J Roentgenol 127:403–407, 1976.
44. Juler GL, Conroy RM, Fuelleman RW: Bile leakage following percutaneous transhepatic cholangiography with the Chiba needle. Arch Surg 112:954–958, 1977.
45. Redman HC, Joseph RR: Hemobilia and pancreatitis as a complication of a percutaneous transhepatic cholangiogram. Am J Dig Dis 20:691–698, 1975.
46. Elias E, Hamlyn AN, Jain S, et al: A randomized trial of percutaneous transhepatic cholangiography with the Chiba needle vs. endoscopic retrograde cholangiography for bile duct visualization in jaundice. Gastroenterology 71:439–443, 1976.
47. Itai Y, Araki T, Yoshikawa K, et al: Computed tomography of gallbladder carcinoma. Radiology 137:713–718, 1980.
48. Raghavendra BN: Ultrasonic features of primary carcinoma of the gallbladder: Report of five cases. Gastrointest Radiol 5:239–244, 1980.
49. Yeh H-C: Ultrasonography and computed tomography of carcinoma of the gallbladder. Radiology 133:167–173, 1979.
50. Yum HY, Fink AH: Sonographic findings in primary carcinoma of the gallbladder. Radiology 134:693–696, 1980.
51. Grank PH, Ridell RH, Feczko PJ, Levin B: Radiological detection of colonic dysplasia (precarcinoma) in chronic ulcerative colitis. Gastrointest Radiol 3:209–219, 1978.
52. American Cancer Society: Guidelines for the cancer related checkup: Recommendations and rationale. CA 30:208–215, 1980.

NINE

Genitourinary Tumors

Ronald A. Castellino and
Garry D. Strauser

The topic "genitourinary tumors" encompasses a variety of tumors within multiple organs. Under consideration in this section are tumors of the urinary tract (kidney, ureter, bladder, urethra), female and male reproductive tracts (uterine cervix and fundus, ovaries with fallopian tubes, vagina, vulva, and prostate, testes, and penis). Within this group occur some of the more common tumors afflicting humans (uterus, prostate, gonads, kidney, and bladder).

This heterogeneous group of tumors does not lend itself to consideration as a unit except in the broadest sense. The following discussion will attempt to approach the consideration of the current state of the art of imaging these tumors, with their advantages and disadvantages, as well as recommendations for future research based on a general evaluation of staging concepts that are broadly applicable to certain of these tumors.

The following discussion will evaluate these tumors in regard to (1) delineation of the local extent of tumor, (2) detection of lymph node metastases, and (3) detection of distant metastases. This follows the generally accepted TNM staging approach and is convenient to use.[1,2] The subsequent discussion will not address itself to imaging methods for the early detection of asymptomatic cancer. The routine radiologic imaging of these various organs under discussion would be extremely time-consuming and expensive and could only be justified if an imaging technique were developed that would detect cancer in an early enough stage to significantly affect morbidity and mortality. Such imaging techniques would probably require detection of disease beyond the resolution of standard imaging procedures; however, nuclear medicine imaging

95

techniques would be appropriate if "tumor-specific" radionuclides were to become available, a discussion left to the chapter on nuclear medicine. In addition, exfoliative cytology for the assessment of uterine cancer has been shown to be effective if conscientiously applied to the patient population. Similar exfoliative techniques might be applied to other organ systems—e.g., cytologic examination of urine, prostatic secretions, etc. Likewise, development of new biologic serum tumor markers (such as those used in testicular cancer) might improve tumor detection. These subjects, however, are outside the scope of this report.

STATE OF THE ART

Delineation of Local Extent of Tumor

Many of the organs under consideration lie within the true pelvis and have certain staging problems in common. Current staging classifications are often related to the extent (depth) of penetration of the tumor into the wall of the organ,[2] a factor that is currently determined on the basis of histologic evidence. This information is probably not readily amenable to radiologic imaging for two reasons: (1) the resolution of imaging techniques in all likelihood will not be able to predict with confidence the level of invasion, which currently is decided by high-power microscopy; and (2) irrespective of how sensitive such imaging techniques become, an initial histologic diagnosis will have to be made—the initial biopsy is planned not only to diagnose the lesion but to establish its histologic stage (e.g., carcinoma of the bladder and cervix).

On the other hand, considerable effort is currently expended to attempt to evaluate the local extent of disease,[3-8] and this area is fraught with inaccuracies.[4,5,9] There is abundant experience in the literature to indicate that the clinical evaluation, which includes the clinical exam and laboratory and radiographic studies, is frequently in error when compared to pathologic staging at the time of subsequent laparotomy or definitive biopsy.[9,10] For example, many prostrate tumors which are felt clinically to be localized to the gland have seminal vesical extension; bladder tumors which are believed to be confined to the bladder wall have perivesical extension.

Current standard imaging techniques in this region include excretory urography, cystography, barium enema examination with or without air contrast, ultrasonography, and computed body tomography. By and large, these modalities provide additional information to the clinical assessment of these tumors but fall short of being reliable to the point of obviating more definitive surgical and pathologic exploration. The latter two techniques—i.e., ultrasound and computed tomography (CT)—are yet in a phase of development. It is hoped that improved resolution and techniques such as CT dynamic mode studies[11] and image reconstruction[3], as described in Chapter 2, will enhance the value of these modalities. The cross-sectional imaging approach of ultrasound and CT lends another dimension to evaluating the extent of tumors within the pelvis, but these modalities lack the fine spatial resolution characteristic of standard roentgenography.

Not included in the above discussion are tumors arising in the testis and kidney–ureter. Evaluation of the local extent of testicular tumors is generally made at the time of orchiectomy where urologic practice indicates that orchiectomy with dissection into the inguinal canal is a preferred method of local staging. Radiologic imaging in this context appears unnecessary. There is, however, the occasional instance in which a patient presents with suspected occult testicular cancer in the presence of known metastatic disease. In this clinical setting, small parts ultrasonographic scanning has been useful in revealing nonpalpable primary tumors.[12] Evaluation of the local spread of renal and ureteral tumors lends itself well to radiologic imaging. The high incidence of renal venous and inferior vena caval invasion with hypernephromas,[13] along with the suboptimal reliability of angiography in staging renal cell carcinoma,[5] should stimulate further interest in evaluation of the ability of noninvasive techniques (such as CT[5,6,13,14] and ultrasound) to detect local extension of neoplasm without having to resort to angiography.

Detection of Lymph Node Metastases

Many of the tumors under consideration have a propensity for lymph node metastases, although some are much more liable to metastasize to lymph nodes than others. In general, the lymph nodes at risk are those that lie along the aorta, vena cava, and the iliac (common, external, internal) arteries and veins and their tributaries, as well as lymph nodes lateral to the paracaval/para-aortic group near the hilus of the kidney.[15] Metastases to lymph nodes situated more anteriorly in the abdomen, such as at the root of the mesentery and along the gastrointestinal tract, are uncommon unless the above-mentioned lymph node groups are involved first. There is ample experience to indicate that evaluation of lymph node metastases by opacification of adjacent organs, as by excretory urography or inferior venacavography, will detect only very bulky disease that is fortuitously placed next to the organ opacified. Lymphography is a much more sensitive indicator of lymph node involvement[16–26] and does not rely upon increased lymph node size to detect metastases. Although it has long been thought that certain critical lymph node groups within the true pelvis which lie along the internal iliac vessels are not opacified by lymphography,[9] more recent work has countered this concept;[27] reproducibility of opacification of these nodes remains to be determined, however. Lymphography does not opacify those nodes which appear to be the first echelon for drainage of testicular tumors near the hilus of the kidneys,[17] and lymph nodes above the level of the second lumbar vertebral body are usually inadequately opacified.[28] Furthermore, lymphography probably requires metastases in the order of 5 mm or more in size before it can convincingly display them,[23] and of course false negatives can result from nonopacification due to complete nodal replacement by tumor.[24] False-positive diagnoses, on the other hand, are related to lymph node infiltration by fat, fibrous tissue, and reactive hyperplasia.[25,26]

CT and ultrasonography has been shown to be especially useful in the evaluation of lymphoma and testicular (particularly seminomatous) tumors and provide an additional approach to lymph node evaluation, as they offer potential for definition of metastases in the internal iliac nodes as well as in the upper para-aortic nodes not usually opacified by lymphography.[28] CT and ultrasonography are noninvasive techniques, a fact which makes them particularly appealing. Since these modalities are not organ-specific, they can also define the primary tumor focus, which is beyond the limits of lymphography.[28] In addition, they can demonstrate nodes that are completely replaced by neoplasm.[24,29] However, ultrasonography and CT currently depend upon the detection of lymph node metastases by an increase in lymph node size, so that, in theory, more false-negative studies will be recorded by CT than by lymphography. With improved resolution and selective imaging agents, perhaps some of this difficulty will be overcome.

It is likely, therefore, that there is no current universal "state of the art" modality for lymph node imaging. While lymphography may yield optimal information in cases where there is little or no nodal enlargement,[28] CT and ultrasonography are likely to be more rewarding in varieties of cancer that cause gross adenopathy.[29,30] Furthermore, a combined imaging scheme is likely to yield optimal information in many cases.[30-35] More extensive prospective, comparative studies are needed.

The use of thin-needle aspiration biopsy, in combination with an appropriate imaging modality, provides additional data for more accurate cancer staging.[24,35,36] This technique is becoming more widely used and has been utilized for restaging in cases of suspected recurrence.[37]

Detection of Distant Metastases

Distant metastatic sites for these tumors include a wide variety of organs, such as the lung, liver, and bones. Improved imaging techniques for these areas will be discussed in other sections. The majority of the tumors under consideration metastasize, not unexpectedly, to the above organs; however, it should be realized that ovarian tumors also have a high propensity for developing peritoneal implants. Evaluation for peritoneal implants is currently performed by cytologically evaluating fluid from the peritoneal space or at surgical exploration. It would be important to develop information regarding the ability of CT and ultrasound to detect small peritoneal implants[38] or to develop techniques such as peritoneography[39] that might outline such sites of metastasis. Otherwise, the detection of distant metastases appears little different from the detection of other tumors under consideration and is discussed in other appropriate sections.

RECOMMENDATIONS FOR RESEARCH SUPPORT

Accuracy of Current Imaging Techniques

Despite some comparative data involving ultrasound versus CT,[40,41] ultrasound versus lymphangiography,[42] and CT versus lymphangiography,[29,31–33,43] there is little solid information available regarding the relative accuracy of various imaging techniques (i.e., IVP, BE, CT, US, LAG) in staging these various pelvic tumors.[33,44] Prospective studies with well designed clinical protocols (1) would answer many of the questions of accuracy and utility of these techniques, (2) should indicate the shortfalls and how they may be overcome, and (3) should also stimulate parallel innovative instrumentation for application to the evaluation of the local extent of these tumors. Such objectives would be best carried out as part of clinical trials in which specific attention is paid to evaluating the diagnostic accuracy of these various imaging modalities. This would require histologic confirmation and would have to be subjected to the rigorous standards of a well designed clinical trial. Participation of multiple institutions and investigators would facilitate collection of an adequate sample size.

   The priority and relevance of this approach is high, since it impacts on decisions being made daily in hospitals throughout the country in regard to patients who are diagnosed as having these tumors. The timetable for development is variable, depending upon the accession rate of patients into the protocols and the statistical breakdown of the findings in order to reach a figure of significance; however, 5 years would seem to be an average time that might be reasonably applied to study of this group. The probability of success is high, since an answer will be forthcoming; on the other hand, the results might not be particularly encouraging, since it seems likely that many techniques will fall short of the accuracy required for application to everyday clinical evaluations of such patients. However, the major sources of error should become apparent and could then be studied more vigorously in an attempt to provide definitive imaging of the local extent of the tumor.

Priority: 1
Duration: 3 to 5 years
Probability of Success: high

Development of Organ-specific Contrast Agents

There is considerable room for improvement in the imaging of the various organs under discussion. For example, although many hollow organs can be opacified for improved delineation of the lumina (e.g., barium gastrointestinal studies, oral cholecystography, and excretory pyelography), "solid" organs by and large do not lend themselves to such enhanced evaluation (evaluation of the liver with Thorotrast was a notable exception, as is the nephrographic phase of an excretory urogram for the kidney). Development of a radiographic contrast agent that would opacify the substance of solid organs (such as the prostate, uterus, and gonads) might provide an avenue for the detection of small lesions and provide the capability for delineating their local extent of disease. Although investigative studies have dealt with opacification of solid structures by direct injection of contrast media into the parenchyma or ductal system of the particular organ (such as the prostate[45] or liver[46]) probably of more practical clinical relevance would be opacification by means of intravenous or oral administration; some such studies have been done with intravenous hepatic- and splenic-specific agents.[47-49] (A possible benefit for such investigation would be in "screening" imaging. For example, if a suitable contrast material could be developed for the prostate, it might detect tumors prior to their causing symptoms or being detectable on a rectal examination. Such an imaging study might then be very useful in the older man who is at high risk for development of prostate cancer.) Such agents would have to be present in a relatively high concentration for depiction by conventional radiography, but, as some studies in this area have shown,[49,50] they could be less efficiently concentrated if imaged by CT. Although CT scanning carries the burden of poorer spatial resolution than is found with conventional radiography, use of CT imaging would thus allow utilization of safer doses with the potential for less toxicity than with previously tested agents and concentrations.[48,49]

Development of *tumor*-specific contrast media[49-51] could become a natural offshoot of this research and could provide another dimension to "screening imaging."

The priority for this task is medium and the timetable for development is unknown, but, with sufficient funds, perhaps preliminary information indicating whether or not this avenue is fruitful to pursue might be available within 3 to 5 years.

Priority: 2
Duration: 3 to 5 years
Probability of Success: moderate to poor

Accuracy of Detecting Lymph Node Metastasis

Although initial studies have been published,[29-33,43] further carefully planned prospective clinical investigations comparing the accuracy of various lymph node imaging techniques (lymphography, CT, ultrasonography) with histologic material should be designed in order to determine which modality is the preferred approach in specific clinical settings. Subsequent investigation should be pursued to improve accuracy by gaining understanding of the causes of false-positive and false-negative diagnoses. The role of nuclear medicine is potentially very exciting, should tumor-specific radionuclides be developed and marketed. The high-density discrimination of CT would make practicable detection of small metastases if a suitable label could be applied to the sites of tumor. Methods should also be investigated to opacify lymph nodes in the deep pelvis (i.e., the internal iliac group) to provide images as seen on conventional lymphography.

The priority and relevance for developing clinical studies is high, since such baseline information is required for everyday clinical practice and would serve as a basis of reference for subsequent investigations in the field. The timetable for development would be approximately 5 years, depending on the accession rate of patients into the protocol. The probability of success is high in developing information, which might not only indicate the inadequacies of existing techniques but also provide specific areas for investigation.

Priority: 1
Duration: 3 to 5 years
Probability of Success: high

Development of New Lymph Node-imaging Agents

A major drawback to the current utilization of lymphography is the need to cannulate a lymphatic channel, which many find difficult and tedious. It would be ideal if a radiographic lymph node contrast agent were available which could be administered more readily, as for instance by subcutaneous injection, and which would opacify lymph nodes with at least as high a degree of resolution as does the currently used contrast (Ethiodol). Some experimental indirect lymphographic agents have been studied, but clinical usefulness has thus far been limited by local inflammatory reaction.[52,53]

The prolonged retention of contrast material by the lymph node is desirable to evaluate the nodes on subsequent serial radiographs but would be of less import if the nodes in question could be readily re-opacified. Another limitation of lymphography is its failure to opacify many of the pertinent lymph node groups. Techniques might be worked out that would be helpful in pelvic tumors (as opacification of mediastinal lymph nodes would be helpful for pulmonary neoplasms). Experimental data indicate that other lymph node groups can be opacified, such as those in the hilus of the liver[46,47] and in the mediastinum[53,54] and those draining the bladder,[55,56] prostate,[57] testes, and uterus.[52] Opacification of lymph nodes in the mesentery and along the other portions of the gastrointestinal tract would be desirable when staging gastrointestinal tumors which have a high propensity for lymph node involvement. If a suitable contrast agent could, for example, be taken orally with sufficient absorption into the lymph nodes, some of these needs might be met.[58]

The priority for such work is medium. Such work would greatly enhance lymph node evaluation by (1) allowing visualization of lymph node groups not seen on conventional lymphography, and (2) facilitating the opacification of lymph nodes once the contrast has disappeared. The timetable for development would probably be at least 5 years and the probability of success only moderate (Table 9-1).

Priority: 2
Duration: 5 years
Probability of Success: moderate

TABLE 9-1. SUMMARY OF PROPOSED PROJECTS

Clinical trials to assess the local extent of tumor in regard to:
   a. Accuracy and utility of various imaging techniques
   b. Shortfalls and how to correct them
   c. Stimulating directed research for improvement in instrumentation and technology
Priority: 1
Duration: 3 to 5 years
Probability of success: high

Development of radiographic contrast agents to opacify solid organs
Priority: 2
Duration: 3 to 5 years
Probability of success: moderate to poor

Clinical trial to evaluate lymph node metastases
  a. Accuracy and utility of various imaging techniques
  b. Shortfalls and how to correct them
  c. Stimulation of directed research for improvement in instrumentation and technology
Priority: 1
Duration: 3 to 5 years
Probability of success: high

Improvement of direct opacification ("lymphography") of lymph nodes
  a. Opacify nodes by less invasive and cumbersome cannulating technique
  b. Opacify nodes not visualized by routine pedal lymphography
Priority: 2
Duration: 5 years
Probability of success: moderate

ACKNOWLEDGMENT

Gratitude is expressed to Dr. P. Ruben Koehler, Department of Radiology, University of Utah, College of Medicine, for review of the original manuscript of this chapter.

REFERENCES

1. American Joint Committee for Cancer Staging and End-results Reporting: Manual for Staging of Cancer, 1978. Chicago, Whiting Press, 1978.
2. International Union against Cancer: TNM Classification of Malignant Tumors, ed 2. Geneva, UICC, 1974.
3. Hamlin DJ, Cockett ATK, Burgener FA: Computed tomography of the pelvis: Sagittal and coronal image reconstruction in the evaluation of infiltrative bladder carcinoma. J Comput Assist Tomogr 5:27, 1981.
4. Hodson NJ, Husband JE, MacDonald JS: The role of computed tomography in the staging of bladder cancer. Clin Radiol 30:389, 1979.
5. Weyman PJ, McClennan BL, Stanley RJ, et al: Comparison of computed tomography and angiography in the evaluation of renal cell carcinoma. Radiology 137:417, 1980.

6. Levine E, Lee KR, Weigel J: Preoperative determination of abdominal extent of renal cell carcinoma by computed tomography. Radiology 132:395, 1979.

7. Winterberger AR, Wajsman Z, Merrin C, Murphy GP: Eight years of experience with preoperative angiographic and lymphographic staging of bladder cancer. J Urol 119:208, 1978.

8. Harada K, Igari D, Tanahashi Y, et al: Staging of bladder tumors by means of transrectal ultrasonography. JCU 5:388, 1977.

9. Novak D, Hilweg D, Haug HP: The role of roentgenographic procedures in staging of carcinoma of the urinary bladder by TNM system. Urol Int 26:149, 1971.

10. Fraley EE, Lange PH, Williams RD, Ortlip SA: Staging of early non-seminomatous germ-cell testicular cancer. Cancer 45:1762, 1980.

11. Young SW, Turner RJ, Castellino RA: A strategy for the contrast enhancement of malignant tumors using dynamic computed tomography and intravascular pharmacokinetics. Radiology 137:137, 1980.

12. Leopold GR, Woo, VL, Scheible FW, et al: High-resolution ultrasonography of scrotal pathology. Radiology 131: 719, 1979.

13. Love L, Churchill R, Reynes C, et al: Computed tomography staging of renal carcinoma. Urol Radiol 1:3, 1979.

14. Smith WP, Levine E: Sagittal and coronal CT image reconstruction: Application in assessing the inferior vena cava in renal cancer. J Comput Assist Tomogr 4:531, 1980.

15. Rouvière H: Anatomy of the Human Lymphatic System, Tobias MJ (trans). Ann Arbor, Mich, Edwards Bros, 1938.

16. Watson RC: Lymphography of testicular carcinoma. Semin Oncol 6:31, 1979.

17. Musumeci R, Pizzocaro G, Farina F, et al: Lymphographic evaluation of 285 testicular tumors. Tumori 60:365, 1974.

18. Wallace S, Jing BS: Lymphangiography in tumors of the female genital system. Radiol Clin North Am 12:79, 1974.

19. Musumeci R, DePalo G, Kenda R, et al: Retroperitoneal metastases from ovarian carcinoma: Reassessment of 365 patients studied with lymphography. AJR 134:449, 1980.

20. Musumeci R, Banfi A, Bolis G, et al: Lymphangiography in patients with ovarian epithelial cancer. Cancer 40:1444, 1977.

21. Kademian MT, Buchler DA, Wirtanen GW: Bipedal lymphangiography in malignancies of the uterine corpus. AJR 129:903, 1977.

22. Johnson DE, Kaesler KE, Kaminsky S, et al: Lymphangiography as an aid in staging bladder carcinoma. South Med J 69:28, 1976.

23. Fuchs WA, Seiler-Rosenberg G: Lymphography in carcinoma of the uterine cervix. Acta Radiol (Diagn) (Stockh) 16:353, 1975.

24. Wallace S, Jing BS, Zornoza J: Lymphangiography in the determination of the extent of metastatic carcinoma. Cancer 39:706, 1977.

25. Spellman MC, Castellino RA, Ray GR, et al: An evaluation of lymphography in localized carcinoma of the prostate. Radiology 125:637, 1977.

26. Kolbenstvedt A: Lymphography in the diagnosis of metastases from carcinoma of the uterine cervix stages I and II. Acta Radiol (Diagn) (Stockh) 16:81, 1975.

27. Merrin C, Wajsman Z, Baumgartner G, Jennings E: The clinical value of lymphangiography: Are the nodes surrounding the obturator nerve visualized? J Urol 117:762, 1977.

28. Roberts KR, Mettler FA Jr.: Diagnostic evaluation of the pelvic and abdominal lymphatic system. Curr Probl Diagn Radiol 8:1, 1979.

29. Ginaldi S, Wallace S, Jing BS, Bernardino ME: Carcinoma of the cervix: Lymphangiography and computed tomography. AJR 136:1087, 1981.
30. Lee JKT, McClennan BL, Stanley RJ, Sagel SS: Computed tomography in the staging of testicular neoplasms. Radiology 130:387, 1979.
31. Dunnick NR, Javadpour N: Value of CT and lymphography: Distinguishing retroperitoneal metastases from nonseminomatous testicular tumors. AJR 136:1093, 1981.
32. Lackner K, Weissbach L, Boldt I, et al: Computed tomographic demonstration of lymph node metastases in malignant tumors of the testicles: Comparison of results of lymphography and computed tomography. ROEFO 130:636, 1979.
33. Kilcheski TS, Arger PH, Mulhern CB Jr, et al: Role of computed tomography in the presurgical evaluation of carcinoma of the cervix. J Comput Assist Tomogr 5:378, 1981.
34. Scheible W, Talner LB: Gray scale ultrasound and the genitourinary tract: A review of clinical applications. Radiol Clin North Am 17:281, 1979.
35. Wallace S, Jing BS, Zornoza J, et al: Is lymphangiography worthwhile? Int J Radiat Oncol Biol Phys 5:1873, 1979.
36. Göthlin JH, MacIntosh PK: Interventional radiology in the assessment of the retroperitoneal lymph nodes. Radiol Clin North Am 17:461, 1979.
37. Dunnick NR, Fisher RI, Chu EW, Young RC: Percutaneous aspiration of retroperitoneal lymph nodes in ovarian cancer. AJR 135:109, 1980.
38. Jeffrey RB: CT demonstration of peritoneal implants. AJR 135:323, 1980.
39. Roub LW, Drayer BP, Orr DP, Oh KS: Computed tomographic positive contrast peritoneography. Radiology 131:699, 1979.
40. Williams RD, Feinberg SB, Knight LC, Fraley EE: Abdominal staging of testicular tumors using ultrasonography and computed tomography. J Urol 123:872, 1980.
41. Nash CH, Alberts DS, Suciu TN, et al: Comparison of B-mode ultrasonography and computed tomography in gynecologic cancer. Gynecol Oncol 8:172, 1979.
42. Hutschenreiter G, Alken P, Schneider HM: The value of sonography and lymphography in the detection of retroperitoneal metastases in testicular tumors. J Urol 122:766, 1979.
43. Zelch MF, Haaga JR: Clinical comparison of computed tomography and lymphangiography for detection of retroperitoneal lymphadenopathy. Radiol Clin North Am 17:157, 1979.
44. Griffin TW, Parker RG, Taylor WJ: An evaluation of procedures used in staging carcinoma of the cervix. AJR 127:825, 1976.
45. Raghavaiah NV: Prostatography. J Urol 121:174, 1979.
46. Burgener FA, Weber DA, Kormano M: Hepatography and liver lymphography by retrograde biliary ethiodol infusion: An experimental study in the dog. Invest Radiol 12:259, 1977.
47. Dumont AE, Martelli A: X-ray opacification of hepatic lymph nodes following intravenous injection of tantalum dust. Lymphology 2:91, 1969.
48. Laval-Jeantet M, Lamarque JL, Dreux P, et al: Hepatosplenography by intravenous injection of a new iodized oily emulsion. Acta Radiol (Diagn) (Stockh) 17:49, 1976.
49. Vermess M, Adamson RH, Doppman JL, Girton M: Computed tomographic demonstration of hepatic tumor with the aid of intravenous iodinated fat emulsion: An experimental study. Radiology 125:711, 1977.

50. Young SW, Muller H, Marincek B: Contrast enhancement of malignant
    tumors after intravenous polyvinylpyrrolidone with metallic salts as deter-
    mined by computed tomography. Radiology 138:97, 1981.
51. Long DM, Multer FK, Greenburg AG, et al: Tumor imaging with x-rays
    using macrophage uptake of radiopaque fluorocarbon emulsions. Surgery
    84:109, 1978.
52. Kaude JV, Abrams RM, Daly JW: Percutaneous indirect lymphography with a
    new experimental contrast medium: A preliminary report. Angiology 29:162,
    1978.
53. Jonsson K, Olin T: The study of iodized oil emulsions for indirect lymphogra-
    phy. Invest Radiol 9:37, 1974.
54. Forsby N, Jonsson K, Olin T: Transabdominal lymphography after intra-
    peritoneal injection of Rous virus in newborn rats. Invest Radiol 13:48, 1978.
55. Böcker R, Huth R: A new method of lymphadenography of the regional
    lymph nodes of the human urinary bladder: Findings relevant to cancer of the
    bladder. Urologe (A) 17:85, 1978.
56. Fiorelli C, Lunghi F, Nicita G, et al: Visualization of paravesical lymphatics
    by direct injection of contrast medium. Urology 11:200, 1978.
57. Raghavaiah NV, Jordan WP Jr: Prostatic lymphography. J Urol 121:178, 1979.
58. Reichel A, Vogler H, Ott J: X-ray contrast presentation of the thoracic duct
    by enterally resorbed iodized oil emulsions in cats and dogs. Lymphology
    3:95, 1971.

TEN

Skeletal System Tumors

Gwilym S. Lodwick

The requirements of bone imaging for the diagnosis and management of cancer are to provide information which allows:

1. The detection of cancer.
2. The display of gross morphology, particularly the location, size, and extent of the tumor.
3. The display of detailed information about the interaction of tumor with bone and soft tissue and about the tumor itself.

From these kinds of information we can learn whether the tumor is localized or disseminated; whether it is confined or has spread to involve vital structures such as vessels, nerves, or organs which may need to be sacrificed in treatment; whether it is slowly or rapidly growing; or whether it is a kind of tumor which must be excised, radiated, or treated by hormones or chemotherapeutic drugs. One would like to learn from imaging as much as possible about the staging of a tumor, Finally, and perhaps most important of all, one would like to learn something about timing of treatment; whether the neoplasm requires immediate attention, whether it can safely be followed for progress, or whether it needs no treatment at all.

Each imaging modality now available to us, including multiple projection radiography, tomography, angiography, xeroradiography, isotope scanning, and computed tomography, has its own special contribution in providing the kind of information needed for the diagnosis and management of cancer. The capabilities of some imaging technologies are well known through experience and time. Roentgen, in 1895, chose radiography of bone for his first experiments. On the other hand, we are now just learning the values of computerized tomography for examination of tumors of the skeletal system and the technique is widely available only in the United States. Our problem is to know the specific merits and weaknesses of each examining modality so as to be able to identify the specific imaging technology (or techniques) most appropriate to solving the specific problem at hand. The strengths and weaknesses of each kind of image are evaluated below and the needs for future investigation are identified.

STATE OF THE ART

Orthogonal Radiography
Multiple projection radiography is generally accepted as the most informative and effective technique for demonstrating gross morphology and fine structure in tumors of bone.[1] Plain radiographs have the capability of spatial resolution of up to 20 line pairs/mm and a density range of nearly three on the H & D curve. Because of this versatility in providing a wealth of detail and contrast for study of a specific lesion, the radiographic examination is mandatory. However, soft tissue extensions in the axial skeleton are difficult to visualize, and tumors arising in spongy bone may not be visible until the cortex is extensively destroyed.[2] Further work is required to develop better high resolution, high speed combinations of films and screens for visualizing fine structures and identifying metastases which cannot be seen with current technology.[3] Combined with magnification radiography, high resolution technologies can enhance detectability of metastatic disease and provide more detailed information concerning the structural alterations associated with tumor progression and regression under therapy.[4,5]

Tomography
Tomography has proved to be of substantial importance in studying gross morphology and fine detail of tumors through elimination of structured noise created by overlying structures. The evidence is clear that tomography provides detail that is important for diagnosis and which is not ordinarily visible on routine films, such as skip areas of disease. Such information often is crucial in deciding whether or not to biopsy. Tomography requires a relatively high radiation exposure, a substantial part of which can be the result of the trial and error test exposures necessary to determine proper technique. Successful modifications of instrumenta-

tion necessary to eliminate or reduce test exposures in number will diminish radiation exposure, time, and costs.

Xeroradiography

The periosteal interface between bone and soft tissue is highly reactive, causing resorption or deposition of new bone in the presence of tumor. Xeroradiography enhances the visualization of these changes, which are difficult to see in film radiography. For this reason, xeroradiography is an important adjunct examination, particularly for the extremities.[6] The value of xeroradiography for bone cancer detection and diagnosis must be considered in any efficacy study.

Arteriography

Arteriographic examinations are often employed in the evaluation of tumors of bone with soft tissue extension, principally because demonstration of the location and displacement of the vessels is helpful in the surgical and radiation therapy management of such lesions. Arteriography provides especially useful information about the soft tissue extent of a primary lesion and occasionally identifies secondary lesions in bone and soft tissue proximal to the tumor.[7] However, arteriography has not been useful in providing information as to whether tumors are benign or malignant or in determining histologic type. It seems likely that computerized tomography will ultimately prove more valuable in evaluating the extension of tumor into soft tissue, particularly in the axial skeleton.

Nuclear Imaging

Technetium-99m (Tc-99m) phosphate scans are essential in the primary evaluation of malignant tumors of bone for determining the presence of additional sites of involvement.[8] In 14 percent of osteosarcomas, metastases appear earlier in bone than in the lungs.[9] Tc-99m phosphate scans are capable of localizing metastatic lesions in the skeletal system which cannot be seen with radiographic techniques. Disadvantages of nuclear imaging are poor spatial resolution and the nonspecific nature of uptake of Tc-99m phosphate. On occasion, metastatic tumors can be seen in x-rays and not in the scans, as with myelomas. There is need to develop quantitative scanning with a scale of densities which can be correlated with different tumors and disorders. Better tumor-specific scanning agents for following the progress of cancer in bone need to be developed for evaluation of the effectiveness of cancer management. Further, tumor-specific scanning agents are needed which can distinguish metastatic from posttraumatic and inflammatory lesions. Emission tomography may prove helpful in diagnosing deep-seated lesions and needs systematic application and evaluation.

Computed Tomography

While orthogonal radiography remains the standard method for examining the gross morphology and detail of tumors in bone, computed tomographic (CT) imaging clearly is superior for the visualization of tumors in the spine, sacrum, and pelvis.[10,11] CT provides excellent demonstration of extension of tumor into the soft tissue and other structures where, even retrospectively, such extensions cannot be detected with standard radiographic imaging. Overlying soft tissues and gas do not compromise the visualization of structure with CT; indeed, with CT, deep structures can be examined through plaster with excellent visualization—an extraordinarily valuable feature.

CT sections are typically in the axial plane, which provides a new perspective and dimension to traditional images or tomograms which are obtained in the sagittal or coronal projections. Multiple parallel CT sections provide the technical feasibility of three-dimensional reconstructions,[12] which delineate surface irregularities and extensions of neoplastic growth and permit more accurate targeting of radiation therapy or better planning of surgical resection. Three-dimensional reconstructed images have not yet been fully assessed and must be systematically evaluated in comparison with other imaging technologies.

An important feature of CT is the potential of developing absolute CT numbers which can be used to accurately identify bone, blood, fluid, and tissue, thus providing additional insight into the morphology of tumors not possible with standard techniques. Such CT numbers are of great potential use for determining the density of bone and the dynamic changes of density which often accompany the presence of neoplasm.[13] A study of the relationship between CT numbers and bone density is important for better understanding of the rate of growth of tumor in bone.

The present disadvantages of CT are the relatively poor spatial resolution as compared with that of traditional radiography, the relatively high radiation exposure entailed, motion artifacts associated with long exposure times, and the cost of equipment. Further technical development is needed to overcome these disadvantages.

Interpretation of Bone Images

Properly interpreted, imaging technologies provide important information about size, shape, extension, and rate of growth which, taken together, can permit a tentative decision about management strategy. Such decisions can be: (1) to do nothing ("leave it alone" lesions), (2) to recommend an immediate biopsy and additional work-up to evaluate possible extension and metastasis, or, in some instances, (3) to establish that a given case falls into a low risk category of disease which can be safely observed to establish its quiescence or for development of additional information.

Given the complexity of this decision process, it is not surprising that the error rate is often 30 percent or greater.[14] With error rates of this order of magnitude, the improvement of human accuracy in diagnosis of bone cancer rates a high priority for support of further research in the diagnostic process.

Research to improve interpretation and decision making also requires the establishment of efficacy studies to determine the relative merits of single or combination imaging technologies in order to determine the most efficacious and cost-beneficial methods of implementing diagnostic and treatment strategies. A natural outcome will be the development of algorithms for clinical decision making, which may be studied as a part of or parallel to application of efficacy protocols.[15,16] Research is also needed for identifying the causes of human error in interpretation of radiant images and the development of interpretative strategies to maximize the usefulness of an examination strategy for the patient and to minimize the risk of poor decisions.

From a global perspective, the values of cancer imaging in bone apply not only to radiologists, but also to orthopedic surgeons, pathologists, oncologists, radiation therapists, and others who accept the responsibility of diagnosis and management of bone cancer. The availability of referral resources for skilled assistance in interpretation of radiographic images and histologic materials is an extremely important part of national effectiveness in the management of bone cancer.

RECOMMENDATIONS FOR RESEARCH SUPPORT

Diagnosis of Cancer: Implementation of Efficacy Studies for Imaging Modalities

Multi-institutional trial studies are needed, with prospective protocols structured to assess the best combinations of film radiography, xeroradiography, film tomography, computed tomography, and radionuclide scanning in tumor diagnosis. These protocols need to be structured to evaluate both primary bone tumors and metastatic lesions. The specific questions which need to be answered concern:

1. Gross tumor morphology (size, shape, and extent).
2. Specific diagnosis and assessment as to whether the tumor is benign or malignant.
3. Rate of tumor growth.
4. Definition of strategy of tumor management (whether to follow the lesion, biopsy, or treat).
5. Assessment of cost, risk, and benefit.

The outcome of these studies should help to determine which of the imaging technologies and combinations of these studies are best for the different tumor locations and for different types of neoplasms and should suggest avenues for future research and development.

Priority: 1
Duration: ongoing
Probability of Success: high

Diagnosis of Cancer: Development of Clinical Algorithms

In an effort to organize, simplify, and standardize the approach to bone tumor diagnosis, research is needed for defining the specific decision pathways for both selection of appropriate imaging modalities and diagnostic tests and subsequent treatment strategies. Decision trees should be developed by panels of experts selected from their respective fields and the results tested with an appropriate protocol and a set of selected test cases. Alternatives to decision trees should be considered. These materials should subsequently be widely distributed to all individuals involved in bone tumor diagnosis.

Priority: 1
Duration: 3 to 6 years
Probability of Success: high

Diagnosis of Cancer: Evaluation of Human
Error in Image Interpretation

To date, no multi-institutional, well controlled study has been applied in the evaluation of the scope of effectiveness for CT with bone tumors both in the axial and appendicular skeleton. The variables which need to be assessed include:

1. The capability of CT to accurately determine gross morphology (size and extent of tumor).
2. The capability of CT to distinguish dense bone, porotic bone (as with permeative bone destruction), soft tissue, blood, and fluid (as in cystic lesions).
3. The capability of CT to accurately reflect the differences between tumor and reactive bone, a major problem in the radiographic interpretation of bone disease.
4. The capability of CT to reflect differences in tumor tissues, particularly textural differences and those indicating the amount of bone, fat, and cartilage within the tumor and contigous bone.

5. The usefulness of combinations of CT with emission tomographic images and/or neutron magnetic resonance images for the correlation of gross morphology and pathophysiologic mechanisms (optional).
6. Further evaluation of the effectiveness of computed tomography in quantifying osteoporosis (optional).

Priority: 1
Duration: 3 to 6 years
Probability of Success: high

Diagnosis and Management of Cancer: Improvement of Diagnostic Quality of Radiographic Images

Comparative evaluations are needed to study the new rare-earth screen–film combinations and magnification radiography with bone neoplasms. Multi-institutional efforts should be directed toward the earlier detection of both primary and metastatic bone lesions. A further objective should be to assess improvements in detail for their impact on both tumor detection and diagnosis, as well as for the assessment of tumor progression and regression. These studies should be fundamental in nature, utilizing information theory as applied to imaging. This research requires the development of detailed information about such factors as effect visibility of tumor in bone, standards for measurement of size of osseous lesions, and the nature of the evidence which indicates progression or regression of metastases.

Priority: 1
Duration: 4 to 6 years
Probability of Success: moderate

Diagnosis of Cancer: Identification of Cancer Behavior in Bone

The ultimate measurement of the effectiveness of any specific cancer therapeutic regime is largely dependent upon being able to observe objective change in tumor behavior. Unlike soft tissue, healing of tumor bone is more difficult to evaluate and often lags radiographically behind the actual biologic responses of the tumor. There is a need for specific studies to permit earlier and more accurate recognition of therapeutic success or failure through observation of radiographic images of both focal and disseminated bone tumors.

Priority: 2
Duration: 2 to 4 years
Probability of Success: moderate

REFERENCES

1. Levine E, Lee KR, Neff J, et al: A comparison of computed tomography and other imaging modalities in the evaluation of musculoskeletal tumors. Presented at the 1978 Scientific Program, Radiology Society of North America, Chicago.
2. Lodwick GS: Reactive response to local imaging in bone. Radiol Clin North Am 2:209–219, 1964.
3. Doi K, Genant HK, Rossman K: Effect of film graininess and geometric unsharpness on image quality, the fine detail skeletal radiography. Invest Radiol 10:35–42, 1975.
4. Genant HK, Doi K: High resolution skeletal radiography: Image quality and clinical application. Curr Probl Radiol 7:1–62, 1978.
5. Logan WW: Breast Carcinoma: The Radiologist's Expanded Role. John Wiley and Sons, 1977.
6. Nessi R, Coopmans de Yoldi G: Xeroradiography of bone tumors. Skeletal Radiol 2:143–150, 1978.
7. Vogeli E, Fuchs WA: Arteriography in bone tumors. Br J Radiol 49:407, 1976.
8. Citron DL, Bessent RG, Grieg WR: A comparison of the sensitivity and accuracy of 99TC^m phosphate bone-scan and skeletal radiography in the diagnosis of bone metastasis. Clin Radiol 28:107–117, 1977.
9. Goldstein M, Zufall E, Jaffin N, Treves S: Changing indications for bone scintigraphy in patients with osteosarcoma, Manuscript under review.
10. Levitt RG, Sagel SS, Stanley RJ, Evens RG: Computed tomography of the pelvis. Semin Roentgenol 13 (3):193–200, 1978.
11. McLeod RA, Stephens DH, Beabout JW, et al: Computed tomography of the skeletal system. Semin Roentgenol 13:235, 1978.
12. Glenn WV Jr, Davis KR, Larsen GN, Dwyer SJ III: Alternative display formats for CT data, in Potchen EJ (ed): Current Concepts in Radiology. St. Louis, C.V. Mosby, 1977, vol 3, pp 88–124.
13. Genant H, Boyd D: Quantitative bone mineral analysis using dual energy computed tomography. Invest Radiol November–December 1977, pp 545–551.
14. Lehr JL, Lodwick GS, Farrell C, et al: Direct measurement of the effect of film miniaturization on diagnostic accuracy. Radiology 118 (2):257–263, 1976.
15. Lodwick GS, Reichertz P: Computer assisted diagnosis of tumors and tumor-like lesions of bone: The limited Bayes' concept. Proceedings of Symposium Osseum, London, April, 1968.
16. Lang EK: Roentgenographic assessment of asymptomatic renal lesions. Radiology 109:257–269, 1973.

ELEVEN

Mammography

John R. Milbrath, James E. Youker,
and Charles R. Wilson

Cancer of the breast represents the number one health concern of the majority of American women. The incidence of breast cancer may be increasing. Today 1 out of every 11 women can expect to have breast cancer in her lifetime.[1] The psychologic impact of mastectomy, the biologic unpredictability of the disease, and the public debate over the theoretic role of radiation in producing breast cancer has resulted in great consternation and confusion among American women.

Early diagnosis remains the best approach to the treatment of this disease. Over a decade ago, the Health Insurance Plan (HIP) of New York study, utilizing what are now antiquated mammographic techniques, demonstrated the ability of screening to improve the mortality rate of breast cancer.[2] The results of the HIP study suggested that screening was only of benefit in women over the age of 50. More recent studies utilizing modern mammographic techniques suggest that women under the age of 50 may also benefit from screening.[3] Mammography can now detect small cancers with very low levels of radiation. For example, in our institution we can now perform mammography at a radiation dose of 35 mR to the midbreast per exposure. Unfortunately, the public concern over radiation has resulted in women avoiding mammography even when they are symptomatic. As a result, many surgeons are now seeing more women with more advanced breast cancer than they did prior to the mammography debate.

Mammography in the symptomatic patient helps to map the tumor for the surgeon or radiation therapist and can discover additional clinically occult breast cancers. There is evidence suggesting that breast cancer is not a focal disease affecting one breast but is part of a generalized disorder.

The treatment of breast cancer, although highly controversial, has undergone considerable change. The classic Halstead mastectomy has been modified, with many women receiving less than a total mastectomy. Radiation therapy is established in the treatment of breast cancer. Furthermore, the use of adjuvant chemotherapy offers promise in extending the life of women afflicted with this very unpredictable disease.

In the last 10 years, radiologists have been provided with powerful tools both for the detection of breast cancer and for the determination of the extent of its spread. One would hope that the medical profession and general public would recognize the progress that has been accomplished and utilize these new methods to effect an earlier diagnosis of breast cancer and, it is hoped, an improved survival rate.

STATE OF THE ART

Diagnosis vs. Screening
A diagnostic examination is done when one has symptoms of a particular disease. The examination is asked to classify each person as either diseased or nondiseased. A screening examination is entirely different in concept. Such an examination is simply asked to to divide a population into two groups, one containing most, if not all, individuals who are likely to have the disease in question, the other consisting of most, if not all, individuals who are unlikely to have the disease.

A low specificity is never acceptable for a diagnostic examination, although it is acceptable for a screening examination—if the sensitivity is sufficiently high.

Until the past few years, mammography was used almost entirely as a diagnostic test. Accuracy in this role was expected to be 90 to 95 percent. However, with the report of the HIP study, mammography began to be utilized more as a screening test.

The results of the Breast Cancer Detection Demonstration Projects (BCDDPs) showed that current mammography is much more effective in detecting cancers, particularly in women under age 50, than it was in the HIP study.[4] In the BCDDPs, about 50 percent of the cancers in screenees were found in women under age 50. Both in women over and women under age 50, about half of the cancers were found on mammography only. A recent review of the mammograms taken during the HIP study showed them to be far inferior in quality to the mammograms obtainable today.[5]

Staging

The stage of breast cancer is assessed by clinical and radiographic methods and then modified on the basis of pathologic results. The TMN classification is based on tumor size, presence or absence of fixation of the tumor to the chest wall, and the presence or absence of axillary nodes or distant metastases.[6]

Stage O cancer is synonymous with minimal breast cancer, as defined by Gallager and Martin.[7] This stage refers to *in situ* cancer or cancer the invasive component of which is 0.5 cm or smaller in size. This stage is regarded as highly curable, with most series reporting 10 year survival of over 90 percent.[8] Stage O cancer can be detected by physical examination but most often is detected by mammography.

Limitations

Dose and Resolution.   It is generally accepted that for early detection of breast cancer, a system must be able to image objects smaller than 0.5 mm in order to detect minute details, such as microcalcifications, changes in the ducts, and the irregular borders frequently seen with cancer. Currently, film–screen systems and xeroradiography meet these criteria and are the two principal systems used for mammography. Nonscreen film, although capable of producing extremely high resolution images with low noise, is not recommended for routine use because of the high radiation dose. A quantitative comparison between film–screen and xeroradiography is extremely difficult, and the choice of one system over the other is at present a subjective matter.

Due to its edge enhancement, xeroradiography provides better visualization of soft tissue details, especially calcifications, than film–screen combinations. The dose to the breast tissue is higher with xeroradiography than with the film–screen systems and, as a consequence, noise is significantly less. Film–screen has a significant dose advantage over xeroradiography and, when the images are not noise limited, film–screen images are diagnostically equal to those obtained with xeroradiography.

Recommendations concerning the appropriate system(s) for mammography have been made by the National Council on Radiation Protection and Measurements (NCRP).[9] According to this report, there is no reason to use molybdenum-tungsten alloy targets. X-ray tubes with tungsten targets and beryllium windows are not to be used unless they meet minimum half-value layer standards; use of these tubes is also not recommended. When using xeroradiography, total filtration in the beam should be equivalent to 2.5 to 3.5 mm of aluminum. Larger amounts of filtration, while further reducing incident skin dose, may lead to higher midbreast doses because of the higher voltage required. Focal spots in the range of 0.5 to 1 mm are to be used when target-to-object and object-to-film distances are reasonable. Minimum target–film distance should not be less than 50 cm. There should be close contact between the breast and the recording medium, and compression devices are desirable. Tube voltages between 25 and 35 kVp are used for film–screen techniques and 35 to 60 kVp for xeroradiography.

Because of the possible carcinogenic effects of radiation, dose to the target tissue should be kept to a minimum without sacrificing clinical information. Radiation exposure at the surface of the breast has been historically used as the measure of the radiation to the patient. However, since it is believed that the tissue at risk is the ductal epithelium, a more appropriate parameter to estimate risk is that of the absorbed dose at midbreast. At present, midbreast doses in xeroradiography are somewhat less than 0.5 rad, while the midbreast dose for film–screen is on the order of 0.1 rad. A mean dose of less than 1 rad should be used in obtaining two views of the breast.[9]

The NCRP has also estimated the risk of developing breast cancer from mammographic procedures. A woman aged 35 who receives 1 rad average midbreast dose increases her life-time natural risk of developing breast cancer from 7.58 to 7.61 percent, or an increase of only 0.03 percent. For an individual, such an increase in risk is insignificant when compared to other risks.[10]

Significant reduction in doses used in film–screen radiography do not appear very likely because at present the images are nearly photon-limited. Further increases in speed of the screen systems would either further increase noise or degrade resolution. Increasing the thickness of photoreceptor used in xeroradiography would reduce the dose, but this would also be expected to cause a decrease in resolution. Plate sensitivity increases with increasing photon energy. However, although increasing the filtration to produce a harder beam would decrease skin exposure, it would also increase the midbreast dose. An immediate 20 to 25 percent reduction in exposure is possible by using negative mode. However, this mode of image presentation has not been generally accepted. Further increases in resolution with film–screen systems are unlikely without sacrificing the present low doses. In xeroradiography, there are indications that direct read-out of the photoreceptor latent image by electronic means, laser interrogation, or other means may lead to increase in resolution and possibly some reduction in dose, but these techniques are still in the investigational stages.

Cost.   Although a mammogram may cost anywhere from $50 to $200, the cost may be considerably reduced in a large volume center. In 1979,

Moskowitz and Fox calculated that the cost of a mammogram at the Cincinnati BCDDP was $10.65.[11] Therefore, even today, a screening examination consisting of physical examination of the breasts and mammography could be performed for less than $25 at a center designed for handling 50 to 100 women per day.

Manpower—Training. It has been estimated that there are not a sufficient number of centers with trained personnel now to screen all women over age 50, even biannually.

If 20 percent of the nation's 50 million women at risk were to desire annual screening, and if each trained radiologist could interpret 20,000 cases/year, then 500 radiologists would be needed. Since mammograms can be done at the rate of 5 women/hour, then using an 80 hour, 2 shift work week, 500 mammographic units would be required.

Mammography is still not a required part of a radiology residency program. However, although still not required, skill in mammographic interpretation is frequently examined during the radiology board examinations. If skill in mammographic interpretation were a requirement of certification, there would be great incentive to make sure all residents were thoroughly trained.

Interventional

Localization. Many of the cancers detected by mammography are nonpalpable. Of the minimal breast cancers found in the BCDDPs, 65 percent were found only by mammography. Prior to the widespread use of localization procedures, 10 to 15 percent of the nonpalpable abnormalities were not removed during biopsy. A localization method is therefore essential to ensure that nonpalpable abnormalities are removed for histologic study.

Various methods for localization are available. Although some use markers positioned on the breast or needles positioned within the breast, we prefer a variation of the "spot" method in which 0.1 cc of a mixture of vital dye and radiographic contrast is injected into the breast.[12]

Specimen Radiography. A radiograph of a biopsy specimen may verify that the nonpalpable lesion has been removed. If the abnormality does not contain calcifications, specimen radiography is of less value.

If the biopsy specimen that contains the nonpalpable abnormality is sliced "bread-loaf" style into sections 2 to 3 mm thick and then radiographed, the radiologist can guide the pathologist in selecting areas to examine histologically.

Specimen radiography is also useful when the entire specimen is so large that it cannot be conveniently examined histologically or when a "blind" biopsy is performed on the contralateral breast.

Biopsy/Aspiration.   Biopsy with subsequent histologic examination is the ultimate diagnostic procedure. If an examination indicates that a particular area of the breast is likely to be cancerous, tissue should be removed for pathologic examination. Radiologists at many centers, including ours, believe that if an abnormality has a 5 percent chance of being malignant, a histologic examination should be done.

Biopsy of a palpable mass may be performed using excisional or incisional technique. Tissue for histologic examination may also be removed by means of needle biopsy techniques.

Cytologic examination may be performed on material obtained on fine needle aspiration. The value of cytologic examination varies from center to center and appears related to the experience of the cytopathologist.

Aspiration is initially performed on most palpable masses. If clear fluid is obtained and the mass disappears, nothing further is done. If clear fluid is obtained but the mass recurs, another aspiration is usually performed. If the mass continually recurs or the fluid is not clear, a biopsy is indicated.

RECOMMENDATIONS FOR RESEARCH SUPPORT

Clinical Studies

Screening.   The value of screening women aged 40 to 49 years must be determined. Although the HIP study failed to show a benefit for screening women under age 50, there are strong indications, particularly from the BCDDP data, that today's mammography is far superior in detecting small, potentially curable cancers.

The report of the Working Group to Review the NCI/ACS Breast Cancer Detection Demonstration Projects recommended as highest priority that the efficacy of screening women aged 40 to 49 be determined.[4]

In addition, they felt that, next in priority, the contribution of mammography in lowering mortality should be determined. HIP showed that the combination of mammography and physical examination reduced the mortality rate, but the independent contribution of mammography was not determined.

The Working Group also felt that annual screening should be compared with biennial screening for women over age 50. The screening in HIP was annual. However, if biennial screening was as effective in reducing the mortality rate, cost and radiation exposure could be effectively reduced.

Priority: 1
Duration: 10 to 15 years
Probability of Success: excellent

Ultrasound. The role of ultrasound in breast disease should be evaluated according to the guidelines recently developed by a subcommittee of the Committee on Mammography of the American College of Radiology.[13] Ultrasound is in the first phase of preliminary evaluation and training. The next phase would be "to determine, in a *blinded* study, whether the device can detect breast lesions presently detectable by the present inplace clinical modalities."[13]

Priority: 1
Duration: 3 years
Probability of Success: moderate

Improved Methods

Electron Radiography and Ionography. Xonics electron radiography (XERG) became commercially available in 1977. The detector is a parallel plate ionization chamber in which x-rays interact with the gas molecules to produce ions. These ions are swept from the chamber by a high electric field and deposited on a plastic imaging foil. The final image is developed by charged liquid toner particles and then laminated. Depending upon the image development parameters, the image contains varying degrees of edge enhancement, while the average midbreast dose is similar to that of film–screen techniques. Resolution is comparable to that of xeroradiography and slightly better than that of film–screen. Noise levels are higher than that of xeroradiography, and present systems are plagued with processing artifacts. Consequently, this system has not gained widespread acceptance. Other ionographic systems are possible, and investigations into the use of liquids and solids for the detector are being pursued.[14] At this point, the sensitivity is quite low, and unless it can be increased significantly, these types of detectors will not be acceptable for mammography.

Further evaluation of the XERG system and further development of other detectors should be encouraged.

Priority: 2
Duration: ongoing
Probability of Success: moderate

Scatter Rejection.   Conventional techniques for rejection of scatter, such as the use of grids and magnification, have been investigated for mammographic application. They have demonstrated increased image contrast which produces increased visibility of microcalcifications and small structures. However, such techniques significantly increase the midbreast dose. The use of a Scanning Multiple Slit Assembly has been recently proposed.[15] This technique is superior in scatter rejection to conventional grid techniques and at the same time provides greater transmission of the primary radiation, which allows a lower dose. Further development of these techniques is necessary.

Priority: 1
Duration: 3 years
Probability of Success: moderate

Innovations and New Ideas

Localization.   A new method for isometric localization of nonpalpable breast abnormalities has recently been devised by Brun del Re et al. [16] The unit, called Isomat, consists of two parallel pieces of plastic supported by a simple metal frame. The upper piece of plastic has a finely perforated grid with metallic reference marks (Fig. 11-1). A craniocaudal view is taken through the perforated grid (Fig. 11-2). A needle is then inserted perpendicular to the lesion. The grid is removed and a mediolateral view is then obtained. The optimum depth of the needle is then determined. This method has proven to be extremely accurate. The unit can also be used to direct a biopsy needle.

Additional improvements in localization techniques may reduce the amount of tissue required on a biopsy.

Priority: 3
Duration: 1 year
Probability of Success: Moderate

Prescreening.   Many attempts have been made to effectively identify which women in the population would benefit the most from screening, particularly mammography, and which women would not benefit since a finding of cancer in them would be extremely unlikely. To date, such attempts have been unsuccessful because the methods are not accurate enough—i.e. do not combine high sensitivity with high specificity.

Even a combination of high risk factors was not felt to be accurate enough to be utilized in determining screening strategy.[17]

Breast parenchymal patterns and thermal signals have recently been advanced as prescreeners, but conflicting results have been reported.[18-21]

Priority: 2
Duration: ongoing
Probability of Success: low

Ultrasound. Ultrasound can accurately separate solid from fluid-filled masses. However, current technology appears limited in the detection of cancer, because of inability to identify small, curable cancers. Ultrasound cannot resolve the small calcifications frequently associated with minimal cancer. This technique appears to have greatest value in the dense breast and therefore may have a role in following younger women with fibrocystic disease.

Research into whether through-transmission scanners may be able to accurately separate benign from malignant tissue, and even characterize benign tissue as either proliferative or bland disease, should be done.

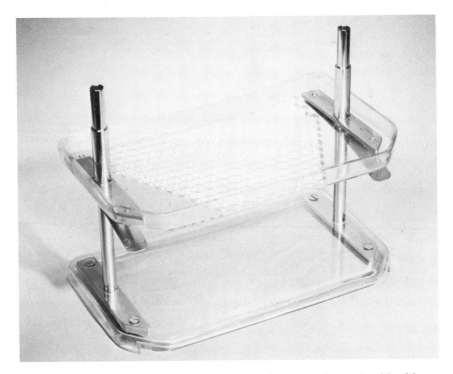

FIGURE 11-1. Isomat grid. The upper plate has a perforated grid with a metallic reference mark.

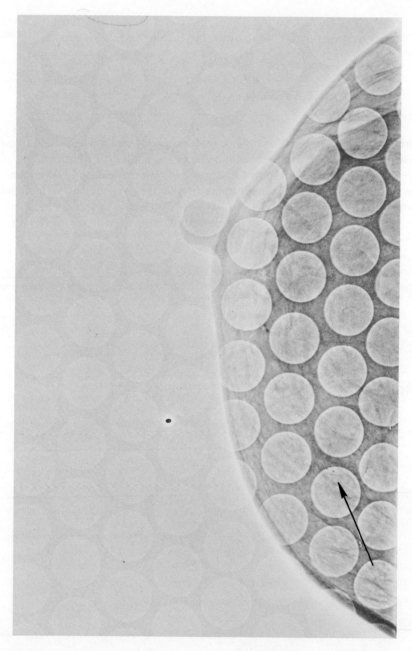

FIGURE 11-2. Localization image. A craniocaudal view is initially obtained and the abnormality is localized (arrowhead marks califications).

Priority: 2
Duration: 5 years
Probability of Success: moderate

Computed Tomography.   Enthusiastic reports by Chang et al. indicate that cancer and premalignant proliferative disease of the breast can cause an abnormal blood–iodine barrier.[22] Thus computed tomography (CT) may identify these areas on a postcontrast scan, even in a dense breast. However, reports from Gisvold et al. are much more cautious.[23] Research in these areas is continuing.

Priority: 2
Duration: 3 to 5 years
Probability of Success: low

Nuclear Medicine.   Lymphoscintigraphy is a simple, nontraumatic, and reproducible technique to evaluate the internal mammary nodes.[24] This technique may aid both the evaluation of possible metastases and radiation therapy planning. Lymphoscintigraphy is presently of little value in axillary lymph node evaluation.

Markers specific for breast cancer or for premalignant proliferative disease have not been found.

Priority: 1
Duration: 3 years
Probability of Success: moderate

Heavy Particle Mammography.   Heavy particle mammography has been used in few centers but apparently can detect the minute differences in density between carcinoma and benign tissue that cannot be detected by conventional mammography.[25] Satisfactory heavy particle mammograms can be produced at radiation doses as low as 100 mR per exposure.

Heavy particles are atoms (usually of carbon, oxygen, or neon) which are stripped of their electrons and accelerated to great energies. Thus this technique suffers the great disadvantage of requiring a cyclotron.

Priority: 3
Duration: 5 years
Probability of Success: moderate

Nuclear Magnetic Resonance. NMR imaging is based on the ability to induce and then monitor the resonance of the magnetic moment of hydrogen nuclei in the presence of magnetic fields. The radiofrequency wavelengths used for imaging and the magnetic fields appear to be completely safe to living organisms. However, its usefulness in detecting breast cancers has not been determined.

Priority: 2
Duration: 5 to 10 years
Probability of Success: moderate

Diaphanography. This is a new update of the old method of transillumination. It is simple and harmless, but its value, particularly in identifying subclinical cancers, has not been determined.

Priority: 2
Duration: 2 to 3 years
Probability of Success: low

Thermography. No method has been more controversial in detecting breast cancers than thermography. Poor results in the BCDDP caused the National Cancer Institute to discontinue thermography as a routine screening test. In 1979, the American College of Radiology and the American Thermographic Society jointly declared that thermography was "not an adequate screening method for the detection of breast cancer or other breast disease when used *alone* or with only a physical examination."[26]

Moskowitz et al. found thermography to be of no greater value than random chance in identifying women with small cancers even if the thermograms were interpreted by recognized experts.[27]

Plate thermography utilizing cholesteric esters has also been proposed as an effective prescreening or even diagnostic method. However, a recent objective study showed plate thermography to be of no value in identifying women with proliferative mastopathy.[28] Therefore, its role as an effective prescreener is in doubt.

Recently, several thermographic units employing computer analysis have been evaluated. The early results are promising, with 80 percent sensitivity *and* specificity.[29] However, its accuracy in identifying women with small cancers has not been determined.

At present, thermography should remain an investigational tool and should not be used in breast cancer screening unless in a scientific protocol.

Thermography has been proposed as a high risk indication. Definite scientific data are, however, lacking. Thermography may have some role in determining a patient's prognosis and therefore therapy, since women with hot thermograms and cancer do not do as well as women with cancer and normal thermograms.[30]

Priority: 3
Duration: 5 to 10 years
Probability of Success: low

Educational Requirements

A recent national survey indicated that mammography training in diagnostic radiology residency programs is less than optimal.[31] Of the programs surveyed, 13 percent did not have personnel with the required training in mammography. According to Homer:

> It is not sufficient for a resident to observe the mammogram being interpreted, and mammography cannot be taught only by formal lectures. The resident must be actively involved in both the supervision and interpretation of the examination. . . .Many residents believe that they are more likely to be shown a case of pseudohypoparathyroidism on their oral boards than a mammogram. If this is true, then the priorities of this certification examination should be re-evaluated. Residency programs will modify the emphasis in their teaching accordingly.[31]

The National Cancer Institute sponsored seven mammography training programs from 1976 to 1979. The programs were discontinued because it was felt that the training belongs in residency programs. However, there are still many practicing radiologists who would benefit from continuing education in mammography. Few fellowships or training programs are available.

In addition, educational programs are needed for the radiologic technologists performing the mammographic examinations. It is our opinion that the quality of mammographic examinations is considerably less than optimal at many centers. This could be changed by educational programs for the mammographer and radiographic technologist.

Priority: 1
Duration: 5 years
Probability of Success: moderate

REFERENCES

1. American Cancer Society, in Cancer Facts and Figures. New York, American Cancer Society, 1980.

2. Shapiro S, Strax P, Venet L, Venet W: Changes in 5-year breast cancer mortality in a breast cancer screening program, in: Seventh National Cancer Conference Proceedings. Philadelphia, J. B. Lippincott, 1973, pp 663–678.

3. Moskowitz M: How can we decrease breast cancer mortality? CA 30:272–277, 1980.

4. Beahrs OH, Shapiro S, Smart C: Report of the Working Group to Review the National Cancer Institute–American Cancer Society Breast Cancer Detection Demonstration Projects. JNCI, 62:641–709, 1979.

5. Gold R: Indications and risk–benefit of mammography. J Fam Pract 8:1135–1140, 1979.

6. Savlov E: Breast cancer, in Rubin P (ed): Clinical Oncology for Medical Students and Physicians, ed 3. Rochester, NY, American Cancer Society, 1970–71, pp 90–104.

7. Gallaher HS, Martin JE: An orientation to the concept of minimal breast cancer. Cancer 28:1505–1507, 1971.

8. Wanebo HJ, Huvos AG, Urban JA: Treatment of minimal breast cancer. Cancer 33:349–357, 1974.

9. Mammography: Recommendations of the National Council on Radiation Protection and Measurements. NCRP Report No. 66, 1980.

10. Feig SA: Benefits and risks of mammography. Presented at the 19th National Conference on Breast Cancer, San Diego, March 9, 1981.

11. Moskowitz M, Fox SH: Cost analysis of aggressive breast cancer screening. Radiology 130:253–256, 1979.

12. Milbrath JR, Shaffer KA, Youker JE: Radiologic detection of breast cancer, in Potchen EJ (ed): Current Concepts in Radiology. St. Louis, C.V. Mosby, 1977, pp 125–142.

13. Moskowitz M, Cole-Beuglet C, Feig SA, et al: The approach to the evaluation of the efficacy of diagnostic imaging procedures for breast disease. Presented at the 19th National Conference on Breast Cancer, San Diego, March 13, 1981.

14. Stanton L: Electrostatic roentgen imaging systems, in Haus AG (ed): The Physics of Medical Imaging: Recording System Measurements and Techniques. New York, American Institute of Physics, 1979, pp 288–304.

15. Yester MV, Barnes GT, King MA: Experimental measurements of the scatter reduction obtained in mammography with a scanning slit assembly. Med Phys 8:158–162,1981.

16. Brun del Re R, Stucki D, Almendral A, Torhost J: A new device for isometric localization of nonpalpable breast lesions detected by mammography, in: IXth World Congress of Gynecology and Obstetrics. Amsterdam, Excerpta Medica, to be published.

17. Farewell VT: The combined effect of breast cancer risk factors. Cancer 40:931–936, 1977.

18. Wolfe JN: Breast parenchymal patterns: prevalent and incident carcinomas. Radiology 131:267–268, 1979.

19. Wolfe JN: Breast patterns as an index of risk for developing breast cancer. Am J Roentgenol 126:1130–1139, 1976.

20. Milbrath JR, Rimm AA: Breast parenchymal pattern and thermographic interpretations as indicators of increased risk for breast cancer. Presented at RSNA, Chicago, November 1977.

21. Moskowitz M, Gartside P, McLaughlin C: Mammographic patterns as markers for high-risk benign breast disease and incident cancers. Radiology 134:293–295, 1980.

22. Chang CH, Sibala JL, Fritz SL, et al: Specific value of computed tomographic breast scanner (CT/M) in diagnosis of breast diseases. Radiology 132:647–652, 1979.

23. Gisvold JJ, Reese DF, Karsell PR: Computed tomographic mammography (CTM). Am J Roentgenol 133:1143–1149, 1979.

24. Ege GN: Internal mammary lymphoscintigraphy: A rational adjunct to the staging and management of breast carcinoma. Clin Radiol 29:453–456, 1978.

25. Sickles EA: Heavy-particle mammography, in Logan WW (ed): Breast Carcinoma: The Radiologist's Expanded Role. New York, John Wiley, 1977, pp 239–241.

26. Schmidt AM, Whitehorn WV, Martin EW: Thermography restriction. FDA Drug Bulletin 6:32, 1976.

27. Moskowitz M, Milbrath JR, Gartside P, et al: Lack of efficacy of thermography as a screening tool for minimal and Stage 1 breast cancer. N Engl J Med 295:249–252, 1976.

28. Moskowitz M, Fox SH, Brun del Re R, et al: The potential of liquid crystal thermography in detecting patients with significant breast mastopathy. Radiology 140:659–662, 1981.

29. Milbrath JR, Schlager KJ: Direct measurement and on-line automatic interpretation of breast thermographs. SPIE–Application of Optical Instrumentation in Medicine VIII 233:282–285, 1980.

30. Gros C, Gautherie M, Bourjat P: Prognosis and post-therapeutic follow-up of breast cancers by thermography, in: Medical Thermography. New York, Karger, 1975, pp 77–90.

31. Homer MJ: Mammography training in diagnostic radiology residency programs. Radiology 135:529–531, 1980.

TWELVE

Childhood Tumors

Herman Grossman and
Carol M. Rumack

In many parts of the world, malignant neoplasms have become second only to trauma as the most common cause of death in childhood. Fewer types of tumors occur in the pediatric age group than in the adult population. Some of these tumors are unique to children. The behavior of some of these tumors is unique as well, including response to treatment. For example, Wilms' tumor, the most comon renal malignancy of childhood, responds to the combined therapy of surgery, chemotherapy, and irradiation in more than 90 percent of the cases of the epithelioid form; renal cell carcinoma, the most common adult renal malignancy, has a less favorable outcome. The 5 year survival of a child with acute lymphoblastic leukemia with combined chemotherapy is more encouraging than the response of an adult patient with leukemia.[1] Solid tumors such as rhabdomyosarcoma[2] and Ewing's sarcoma[3] show great promise for successful responses to combined therapy regimens. However, neuroblastoma, a solid tumor occurring primarily during childhood, has a very poor response to therapy.[4] Under 1 to 2 years of age, the prognosis with neuroblastoma is good because of spontaneous regression of the tumor. Non-Hodgkin's lymphomas in childhood respond much less well to therapy than do the malignancies in adults with this group of diseases.[5]

The histopathology, natural history, and pathways of dissemination and the responses to surgical, radiotherapeutic, and chemotherapeutic management of childhood malignancies have been thoroughly studied. An area of pediatric oncology that has not been well documented is the efficacy of obtaining several types of diagnostic imaging studies in each patient. In general, the following areas need to be more closely defined:

131

(1) evaluation of the type of imaging procedure best suited for the initial detection of the pediatric neoplastic process; (2) evaluation of the appropriate imaging studies required to stage; (3) recommendation of procedures best suited for the detection of distant metastatic disease; and (4) selection of procedures appropriate to the assessment of complications of treatment.

Too often children are subjected to imaging procedures that will not influence their management. Nor do many of these add to scientific knowledge when investigative studies are not part of a cooperative study or when the imaging procedure used has not yet been analyzed for efficacy. A few examples include doing "routine" radioactive isotope bone scans *and* roentgenographic skeletal surveys for patients with neuroblastoma, non-Hodgkin's lymphomas, and rhabdomyosarcoma; evaluating the skeleton in leukemia; and performing radioactive isotope scans of the liver and spleen in Wilms' tumor.

Guidelines will be suggested for imaging modalities for pediatric malignancies, and some suggested protocols for investigative proposals will also be presented.

The recommended protocols described in this report are only recommended. They are based on the best we can derive from clinical experience and the literature. Such protocols cannot be made definitive until we adopt an integrated approach to diagnosis. Pediatric oncologists and other physicians in subspecialties that relate to neoplastic diseases in children must be invited to join pediatric radiologists in panel discussions to decide which of these traditionally performed tests are justified. In many cases, the need for investigative and comparative studies will become clear. The recommended protocols and studies for investigative consideration proposed in this chapter constitute reasonable working outlines to which study groups of specialists can react. The first underlying assumption of this report, therefore, is that all investigative studies and officially recommended protocols should be based on the combined expertise and experience of pediatric oncologists, pediatric radiologists, pediatric surgeons, radiotherapists, and other physicians involved in the management of children with cancer.

A second underlying assumption of this report is that all investigative studies will be cooperative, drawing patient material from several institutions. Cancer is rare in children and a study limited to a single institution would take far too long to complete.

Children with suspected tumors are often subjected to too many radiologic tests. Many of these contribute little or nothing to arriving at a correct diagnosis or assessing the extent of the disease. We can limit the number of tests if we know where and at what age the cancer usually appears; if we know about the various types of a single cancer; if we know the incidence of rapid metastasis in individual diseases; and if we know what organs are likely to be affected when a disease spreads. It is just as important that we have a clear idea of the limits, capabilities, promises, and risks of imaging tools available. The final protocols and associated investigative and comparative studies will reflect a deepening understanding of the diseases, changes in accepted treatment regimens, and developments in the radiologic imaging field. The rational, integrated approach to radiologic study of children with suspected tumor should be a great improvement over our present methods and would establish the format and flexibility needed to respond to developments in cancer research and radiologic imaging.

One approach to all abdominal and pelvic masses in children would be to *start with ultrasonography*, which would determine whether the mass is extra- or intrarenal and whether it is cystic or solid. After 1 year of age, solid renal masses are usually Wilms' tumors; from infancy to about 5 years of age, solid adrenal and paravertebral masses are due to neuroblastoma. These two tumors constitute the majority of abdominal solid tumors in childhood.

If the renal mass is cystic, it will almost always be a benign lesion.[6] The excretory urogram and/or the radioactive isotope scan will define those portions of the kidney which are functioning. Newborn infants may require isotope scans due to the typical poor renal function in the first weeks of life. Cystic abdominal masses usually do not need further preoperative evaluation because they are rarely malignant in children. In the rare instance that a lesion such as a purely cystic neuroblastoma is removed, metastatic evaluation can be done postoperatively.

If a renal mass is found to be solid by ultrasound, computed tomography with enhancement is recommended.[7,8]

STATE OF THE ART

Wilms' Tumor

Wilms' tumor, also known as nephroblastoma, is the most common renal malignancy of childhood. Although the lesion is seen in older children and occasionally in adults, approximately 90 percent of Wilms' tumors occur in patients who are under 8 years of age. The average age at which the tumor is recognized is 3 years. Wilms' tumors make up approximately 10 percent of all childhood malignancies.[9]

Wilms' tumor can be divided into favorable and unfavorable forms by histologic characteristics.[10] Predominantly epithelial tumors with well formed glomerular structures and tubules have a better prognosis than those in which undifferentiated spindle elements (sarcomatous and anaplastic cells) predominate. Research into the latter form of Wilms' tumor should be directed toward evaluation of the therapeutic regimen and refinement of diagnostic accuracy. The recommendations below apply equally to the epithelioid form of Wilms' tumor and the anaplastic and sarcomatous type.

When Wilms' tumor metastasizes, it most frequently does so to the lungs. Metastatic Wilms' to the skeleton is uncommon, but when it does occur it is probably more common in those patients with the sarcomatous type of Wilms'.

Recommended Work-up for Initial Evaluation of Wilms' Tumor

ULTRASONOGRAPHY. Ultrasonography is very helpful in determining if a mass in the kidney is a solid tumor, which in the pediatric age group is assumed to be a Wilms' tumor. The ultrasonogram of patients with Wilms' tumor demonstrates echoes, indicating a solid tumor. Hemorrhage and necrosis, which are often present, produce a mixed pattern of echoes and echo-free areas. Approximately 10 percent of patients with Wilms' tumor have extension into the renal vein and inferior vena cava, almost always arising from tumors in the right kidney (90 percent of cases). Ultrasound can be used to detect tumor extension into the vena cava;[11,12] ultrasound obtains better visualization of the more proximal portion of the cava than is obtained with computed tomography (CT). Metastasis to the liver is uncommon at the time of initial diagnosis. Ultrasound and CT are adequate for evaluating the liver.

BODY CT WITH ENHANCEMENT. Body computed tomography with enhancement can determine whether the tumor has extended beyond the capsule, information that is important for staging. CT has also demonstrated lesions in the opposite kidney that were not seen on excretory urograms, with ultrasound, or at surgery.[13] CT also aids in the assessment of the renal fossa and adjacent tissues, the liver, and the inferior vena cava. CT with enhancement should differentiate intrinsic tumor in the cava from extrinsic pressure. [14-16] At the conclusion of the CT, computer reconstruction or an abdominal roentgenogram will demonstrate the excretory urographic phase of this study. The computed tomographic study of the body should include chest CT as the primary modality to rule out metastatic disease to the lungs.[17-20] Utilizing the technique of representative CT number reported by Siegelman et al.,[21] malignant disease can potentially be separated from the higher density benign lesions. CT would thus allow staging of the primary tumor and assessment of the chest, inferior vena cava, liver, and surrounding structures. The approach does promise cost efficacy.

CHEST ROENTGENOGRAMS. These include frontal and lateral chest roentgenograms or, preferably, stereoscopic views in the frontal projection and a lateral view.

EXCRETORY UROGRAM. If urography is done, the radiographic feature of the disease is displacement and distortion of the pyelocalyceal system. The 5 to 10 percent of cases in which the collecting system is not visualized are associated with extension of tumor into the renal vein, obstruction of the renal pelvis or ureter, or replacement of renal tissue with tumor.[9] Total body opacification is an unreliable tool for finding Wilms' tumor because lucent areas may represent hemorrhage and necrosis in a solid tumor or a benign cystic lesion. If this examination is done, inferior vena cavography should be performed as part of the study. The injection of contrast material should be in a foot vein, and serial roentgenograms should be obtained utilizing 105 mm filming.

ARTERIOGRAPHY. Arteriography has not aided in the staging or management of the disease in children with Wilms' tumor.

Neuroblastoma (Abdominal and Pelvic)
The peak incidence of neuroblastoma is at 2 years of age or younger, with approximately three-fourths of all tumors occurring during the first 4 years of life. As spontaneous regression in infants under 1 year of age with neuroblastoma is "frequent," the impact of various treatment regimens is difficult to assess. In older patients, treatment with chemotherapy and/or radiation therapy in conjunction with surgery has not appeared to improve survival. As most of these patients present with widespread disease, the primary imaging obligation is to assess the extent of disease, primarily within the liver, central nervous system (CNS), and skeleton. CT is an effective imaging modality for determining extent in the abdomen, pelvis, and CNS. Sedation is usually required for accomplishing a satisfactory study. Ultrasonography for abdominal and pelvic neuroblastoma may be satisfactory for following patients. This examination is less expensive, requires no sedation, and often is done in a shorter period of time.

Recommended Work-up for Initial Evaluation of Abdominal Pelvic Neuroblastoma

ULTRASONOGRAPHY. On ultrasonography, neuroblastoma is usually echoic, although homogenicity of neuroblastoma tissue may occasionally produce an anechoic pattern.[22] Evidence of metastases in the liver can be detected by ultrasonography.

EXCRETORY UROGRAM. If ultrasonic identification of the mass as adrenal is uncertain, then an excretory urogram will frequently reveal downward displacement of the kidney. Occasionally the adrenal gland is anterior to the kidney and has no effect on the kidney.[9]

EVALUATION OF METASTASES. Radioactive isotope studies often reveal skeletal metastases earlier than roentgenograms.[23] Because of frequent symmetric metaphyseal metastases, the bone scan may be difficult to interpret and bone roentgenography will be necessary.

In spite of the relative lack of fat in children, preliminary CT studies show good delineation of the primary site of the neuroblastoma and its effect on adjacent tissues. Fast scanning units with improved resolution should make this technique more easily applied and should make the yield higher for determining local extent and lymph node, liver, and adjacent bone involvement. For follow-up evaluation of therapy, CT is more consistently accurate than ultrasound, but the latter modality may be satisfactory.

Neuroblastoma (Thoracic, Posterior Mediastinum)

A posterior mediastinal mass in the pediatric age group most commonly represents a neural tumor. Benign ganglioneuroma represents the most frequent differential diagnosis with malignant neuroblastoma in this region.

Recommended Work-up for the Initial Evaluation of Thoracic Neuroblastoma

1. Chest roentgenograms in the posterior–anterior (P–A) and lateral views.
2. Spine series, including frontal, lateral, and both oblique views in the area of the tumor.
3. Myelography.[24]
4. Computed tomography of the spine in the area of the tumor.[25]
5. Skeletal survey using radioactive isotope scanning.
6. Excretory urography and abdominal ultrasound.

If no disease is demonstrated below the diaphragm, then liver nuclear scanning may be necessary.

Bone Tumors[26–28]

The primary malignant tumors of bone occurring during childhood are, in order of frequency, osteosarcoma, Ewing's tumor, primary lymphoma of the bone, fibrosarcoma, chondrosarcoma, and juxtacortical osteosarcoma.

In the first 5 years of life, malignant bone tumors are exceedingly rare. From the age of 5 to 10 years, the incidences of Ewing's sarcoma and osteosarcoma are about equal. During the second decade of life, osteosarcomas reach their peak incidences and are more frequently reported than Ewing's sarcoma. As age increases, Ewing's sarcoma of flat cancellous bone becomes increasingly more common than Ewing's sarcoma of tubular bone. This discussion will consider osteogenic sarcoma and Ewing's sarcoma of the tubular bones only.

Radiologists should have three objectives in imaging malignant bone tumors: (1) definition of the extent of the primary disease, particularly intramedullary extension and soft tissue extraosseous tumor component; (2) definition of tumor extent (skip areas, multifocal skeletal lesions and/or lung metastases; and (3) follow-up. As all primary bone tumors spread to the lungs and many spread to the skeleton, imaging techniques that assess these areas most efficiently need to be employed.

Recommended Work-up of Primary Bone Tumors

1. Roentgenograms of the involved extremity in multiple projections.
2. Computed tomography of the involved bone.[16,29]
3. P–A and lateral chest roentgenograms and, when possible, stereoscopic chest views. If the latter technique is not available, shallow oblique views should be obtained.
4. Computed tomography of the lungs, mediastinum, and bony thorax.[18,19]
5. Radioisotopic bone scans and radiographic bone surveys should be obtained before initiation of systemic chemotherapy.
6. Protocols for follow-up chest roentgenograms of treated patients without metastasis are under constant review and revision so that no dogmatic recommendation can be made. However, 75 percent of metastases and recurrences occur within the first 2 years following cessation of therapy. It is during this period of time that close evaluation of the lungs for metastasis is necessary.

Hodgkin's Disease[30,31]

Hodgkin's disease is rarely, if ever, seen before the age of 1 year. From age 4 years on, its incidence steadily increases to a first peak in the third decade of life. The histopathologic hallmark of Hodgkin's disease is the presence of Reed–Sternberg cells. In addition, four major histologic types can be identified: lymphocyte predominance, nodular sclerosis, mixed cellularity, and lymphocyte depletion. The choice of treatment for Hodgkin's disease depends upon the histologic type, stage of disease extent, and the age of the patient. Radiation therapy plays a key role, and chemotherapy has become increasingly important in the treatment of Hodgkin's disease in children.

The nodular sclerosis form of Hodgkin's disease is the most common histologic type in children, followed by the mixed cellularity type. The lymphocyte depletion form of this disease is very uncommon in childhood. The survival rates for nodule sclerosis, mixed cellularity, and lymphocyte depletion are similar in the adult and the child when treated in a similar manner.

Current Recommended Work-up for Hodgkin's Disease

CHEST ROENTGENOGRAMS. These include P–A and lateral views for evaluation of intrathoracic lymph nodes, lungs, pleura, heart, and pericardium, as well as the bony thorax. The internal mammary chain of lymph nodes is best seen on the lateral chest roentgenogram.

FULL LUNG TOMOGRAPHY. If the chest roentgenogram contains an abnormal or equivocal finding, tomography may demonstrate hilar lymphadenopathy when the hilae are obscured by a large mediastinal mass on chest roentgenograms. The tomograms may also resolve the question of whether a density seen on the chest roentgenograms represents a disease process or a normal thymus.

CT SCANNING WITH ENHANCEMENT. Utilization of a breath-holding scanner should be the method of choice for studying lymphadenopathy in the abdomen.[32,33] If there are no enlarged nodes, lymphangiography should be considered. Chest CT may eventually replace full-lung tomography for hilar adenopathy, in addition to its use for peripheral metastases.

PEDAL LYMPHANGIOGRAPHY. If retroperitoneal lymphadenopathy is not demonstrated by CT, then lymphangiography can be considered an option, since this is the most direct method for roentgenographically visualizing the parailiac and paralumbar lymph nodes. This modality (1) permits suspicion to be raised concerning lymph nodes that are normal in size, guiding the choice of which lymph nodes to biopsy by laparotomy for staging the disease; (2) provides the radiation therapist with treatment fields; and (3) aids in assessing the response of the disease to therapy.

Non-Hodgkin's Lymphoma

The non-Hodgkin's lymphomas are a heterogeneous group of disorders with varying histologic findings, clinical presentations, and modes of spread. All forms of the disease in children take a rapid course and carry a high mortality. Unlike Hodgkin's disease, the clinical expression of non-Hodgkin's lymphomas in the adult population is quite different from that encountered in children. The most common subtype in childhood is diffuse undifferentiated non-Burkitt's lymphoma.[34]

The detailed anatomic staging information sought in Hodgkin's disease is often not needed in children with non-Hodgkin's lymphoma, because many of these children have widespread, advanced disease at the time of diagnosis.

Rhabdomyosarcoma

Rhabdomyosarcoma is the most common soft tissue sarcoma that occurs in infancy and childhood. Of the solid tumors, its incidence is exceeded only by brain tumors, neuroblastoma, and Wilms' tumor. The tumor can be classified into four histologic categories. The embryonal form is the most common in the pediatric age group and has the best prognosis. The sarcoma botryoides is a type of embryonal rhabdomyosarcoma with a distinctive grape-like polypoid appearance; it is seen most commonly in tumors of the genitourinary tract. The alveolar form occurs primarily on the extremities in older children and is considered to have the poorest prognosis. The pleiomorphic form originates primarily on the trunk or the extremities in adults and is uncommon in children. The two most common sites of rhabdomyosarcoma are the head and neck[35] and the genitourinary tract.[36]

Recommended Work-up for Head and Neck Rhabdomyosarcoma

SUPERFICIAL TISSUES

1. Skull roentgenograms. Bone x-rays of the underlying soft tissue should be examined with skull roentgenograms.
2. Computed tomography. If there is any question of involvement of the bones of the skull, then computed tomography should be performed. This modality will give information about the soft tissues as well as the bony structures.[37]
3. Sialography should be performed if there is a possibility that there is a mass in the parotid.

ORBIT OF THE HEAD AND NECK LESIONS

1. Computed tomography. The bony orbit is a common site for rhabdomyosarcoma.[38] Metastases to the lymph nodes in this region or to distant sites are uncommon due to poor lymphatic drainage within the orbit. Invasion of the tumor locally into the central nervous system, not metastasis, causes death. Skull and facial bone examina-

tion generally reveals no obvious bone destruction. CT is useful for detecting early bone changes and extraorbital extension.

2. Cerebral angiography. Cerebral angiography can demonstrate the abdominal blood supply of the intracranial extension of the tumor.

NASOPHARYNX AND PARANASAL SINUSES. The tumor mass may cause symptoms due to local obstruction. It is also probable that the tumor will metastasize. There is rich lymphatic drainage in this area and the tumor metastasizes to regional lymph nodes early and invades contiguous tissue, causing extensive bony destruction.[39]

The skull and facial bones may be eroded by the expanding tumor, often into the cranial vault. Invading tumor can also cause deformities of soft tissue planes.

CT should be done in all of these patients to demonstrate the extent of bony destruction and invasion by the tumor mass, most frequently into the cranial vault. Angiography is not routinely employed because complete surgical excision of the tumor is not possible.

MIDDLE EAR AND EXTERNAL AUDITORY CANAL. In childhood, rhabdomyosarcoma is the most common neoplasm of the middle ear and external auditory canal. The prognosis for children with rhabdomyosarcoma in this location is very poor, because the tumor causes extensive destruction as it extends into the floor of the posterior cranial fossa and medial cranial fossa and as it expands anteriorly into the sphenoid bone.

1. Skull and mastoid x-rays.
2. Hypocycloidal tomography. Destruction can be seen on skull and mastoid roentgenograms; hypocycloidal tomography defines the petrous bones more accurately.
3. With the newer computed tomographic units fine bone detail can be obtained, and in addition, soft tissue extent and intracranial extension of tumor can be detected. In this way the need for hypocycloidal tomography can be eliminated.

Recommended Work-up for Pelvis Rhabdomyosarcoma

1. Excretory urography with inferior venacavography obtained in the early phase of the study.
2. Ultrasonography.
3. Computed tomography with enhancement.

In evaluating the extent of tumor size in the pelvis, combined inferior venacavography and excretory urography have previously been the method of choice. With good quality CT and ultrasound, a barium enema would not be likely to add any additional data. Of course, abdominal CT might require a gastrografin enema to rule out pelvic involvement adjacent to the colon, but this could be obtained as part of the original CT. Ideally, ultrasound would replace CT, but there are many artifacts in the midabdomen from bowel gas. Ultrasound may be the best modality in very thin patients with very poor tissue plane separation due to lack of fat. CT is the best modality in children with adequate fat planes.

Combined efficacy studies by multiple institutions should eventually determine the final best approach.

Recommended Work-up for Rhabdomyosarcoma of the Extremities. Rhabdomyosarcoma of the extremities is more common in the lower extremities and most frequently occurs in late childhood. The soft tissue mass is usually the first complaint. Metastases occur early to regional lymph nodes. Tumors of the lower extremities metastasize to the abdomen and lungs twice as frequently as tumors of the upper limb extremities. It is rare to have bony involvement with soft tissue rhabdomyosarcoma of the extremities.

Metastases to regional lymph nodes and intraabdominal spread, as well as metastases to the lungs, bone, brain and other structures, appear to be more prevalent in this group of patients than in patients with the other forms of rhabdomyosarcoma. Therefore, initial evaluation should include searching for possible spread to the above-named organs.

1. Chest roentgenograms in the P–A and lateral projections as well as stereoscopic views (or shallow oblique views when stereoscopic views cannot be done) should be obtained.
2. Full-lung tomography and/or computed tomography should be limited to those patients with suspicious areas on the chest roentgenograms.
3. Skeletal studies using radioactive isotope scanning.
4. CT of the head for intracranial and cerebral metastases. Computed tomography is the modality of choice for screening these patients.

RECOMMENDATIONS FOR RESEARCH SUPPORT

Investigative Consideration: Abdominal–Pelvic Neuroblastoma

Liver–Spleen Radionuclide Scintigraphy in Comparison with Ultrasound and CT. Since cures are uncommon in children with neuroblastoma, the purpose of imaging in these patients is to evaluate the various modes of therapy that are tried. Metastases to the liver is common in neuroblastoma. Comparison studies are recommended to see if liver–spleen radionuclide scintigraphy can be eliminated and if CT can be used in a more limited manner, with ultrasound becoming the more routine follow-up modality.

Priority: high
Duration: 3 to 4 years
Probability of Success: high

Comparison of Radionuclide Bone Scans and Skeletal Radiography. Since the skeleton frequently is involved with neuroblastoma, comparison of the medial imaging devices is essential. Controlled, comparative, multi-institutional studies evaluating these two techniques have not yet been done, comparing not only the presence of metastatic osseous lesions and the sensitivity of the imaging modalities, but also the patient's symptoms.

Priority: high
Duration: 3 to 4 years
Probability of Success: high

Investigative Consideration: Bone Tumors
The three objectives for imaging malignant bone tumors set forth earlier in this chapter need to be evaluated to see what influence they have had in patient planning (disarticulation versus limited amputation, various chemotherapy regimens, etc.). This evaluation may show that certain studies can be eliminated (radioisotopic bone scans and/or bone surveys, etc.).

Priority: high
Duration: 3 to 5 years
Probability of Success: high

Investigative Consideration: Hodgkin's Disease
Neither liver–spleen radioisotope scanning nor radionuclide bone scanning in the newly diagnosed patient yields enough new information to justify further investigation. Since most patients undergo exploratory laparotomy, tissue from the liver and spleen will be available for the more definitive histologic analysis.

Computed Tomography of the Lung. Computed tomography of the lung should be done in those patients undergoing full-lung tomography. Both methods can be used to assess involvement of specific nodes in this region.

The study could be completed in 2 to 3 years, with a good probability of obtaining a definitive answer to whether CT should completely replace tomography or is complementary. A moderate priority should be attached to this study because the findings are not likely to change the treatment of these patients.

Priority: moderate
Duration: 2 to 3 years
Probability of Success: high

Abdominal CT. CT of the abdomen can give information about adenopathy and involvement of the liver and spleen. If we assume the patient is going to have a laparotomy, the role of lymphangiography should be raised. Comparison of these two modalities would help answer whether the latter study can be eliminated or whether the examinations are complementary.

The problem of metallic surgical clips used at biopsy sites at the time of laparotomy must be considered if CT is to be utilized for follow-up in those patients with abdominal adenopathy. Plastic clips should be developed which could be seen on CT and possibly on abdominal films but without the very high density, which causes severe artifacts on CT.

Priority: high
Duration: 2 to 3 years
Probability of Success: high

Investigative Consideration: Rhabdomyosarcoma

The need for CT, vascular, or lymphangiography procedures for pelvic or retroperitoneal metastases should be evaluated before undertaking studies of these invasive procedures.

Skeletal survey and liver–spleen scans are generally recommended (in addition to radiographic examinations planned on the basis of the organ of involvement) in patients with all forms of rhabdomyosarcoma. Therefore, it would be worthwhile to look at all skeletal surveys, liver–spleen scans, and chest roentgenograms for rhabdomyosarcoma in all portions of the body to see whether the incidence of distant disease at the time of diagnosis warrants their continued use as routine examinations.

Priority: high
Duration: 5 years
Probability of Success: high

ACKNOWLEDGMENT

The authors wish to thank Mrs. Jacqueline D. Wright for her assistance in the preparation of this chapter.

REFERENCES

1. George SL, Fernbach DJ, Vietti TJ, et al: Factors influencing survival in pediatric acute leukemia: The SWCCSG experience, 1958–70. Cancer 32:1542–1553, 1973.
2. Ortega JA, Rivard GE, Issacs H, et al: The influence of chemotherapy on the prognosis of rhabdomyosarcoma. J Med Pediatr Oncol 1:227–234, 1975.
3. Pritchard DJ, Dahlin DC, Dauphine RT, et al: Ewing's sarcoma: A clinico-pathological and statistical analysis of patients surviving five years or longer. J Bone Joint Surg [Am] 57:10–16, 1975.
4. Sutow WW, Gehan EA, Heyn RM, et al: Comparison of survival curves 1956 vs. 1962, in children with Wilms' tumor and neuroblastoma. Pediatrics 45:800–810, 1970.
5. Murphy SB, Frizzeva G, Evans AE: A study of childhood non-Hodgkin's lymphomas. Cancer 36:2121–2131, 1975.
6. Haller JO, Schneider M, Kassner EG, et al: Sonographic evaluation of mesenteric and omental masses in children. AJR 130:269–274, 1978.
7. Berger PE, Munschauer RW, Kuhn JP: Computed tomography and ultrasound of renal and perirenal diseases in infants and children: Relationship to excretory urography in renal cystic disease, trauma and neoplasm. Pediatr Radiol 9:91–99, 1980.
8. Brasch RC, Abols IB, Gooding CA, et al: Abdominal disease in children: A comparison of computed tomography and ultrasound. AJR 134:153–158, 1980.
9. Grossman H: Evaluating common intra-abdominal masses in children: A systematic roentgenographic approach. CA 26 (4):219–233, 1976.
10. Beckwith JB, Palmer NF: Histopathology and prognosis of Wilms' tumor: Results from the First National Wilms' Tumor Study. Cancer 41:1937–1948, 1978.
11. Goldstein HM, Green B, Weaver RM: Ultrasonic detection of renal tumor extension into the inferior vena cava. AJR 130:1083–1085, 1978.
12. Taylor KJW: Ultrasonic investigation of inferior vena caval obstruction. Br J Radiol 48:1024–1026, 1975.

13. Grossman H, Korobkin M, Kirks DR, Breiman RS: Bilateral Wilms' tumor: Utilization of computed tomography. To be published.
14. Berger PE, Kuhn JP: Computed tomography of tumors of the musculoskeletal system in children. Radiology 127:171–175, 1978.
15. Brasch RC, Korobkin M, Gooding CA: Computed body tomography in children: Evaluation of 45 patients. AJR 131:21–25, 1978.
16. deSantos LA, Goldstein HM, Murray JA, Wallace S: Computed tomography in the evaluation of musculoskeletal neoplasms. Radiology 128:89–94, 1978.
17. Heitzman ER: Computed tomography of the thorax: Current perspectives. AJR 136:2–12, 1981.
18. Kirks DR, Korobkin M: Chest computed tomography in infants and children: An analysis of 50 patients. Pediatr Radiol 10:75–82, 1980.
19. Muhm JR, Brown LR, Crowe JK, et al: Comparison of whole lung tomography and computed tomography for detecting pulmonary nodules. AJR 131:981–984, 1978.
20. Schaner EG, Chang AE, Doppman JL, et al: Comparison of computed and conventional whole lung tomography in detecting pulmonary nodules: A prospective radiologic–pathologic study. AJR 131:51–54, 1978.
21. Siegelman SS, Zerhouni EA, Leo FP, et al: CT of the solitary pulmonary nodule. AJR 135:1–13, 1980.
22. Yeh HC, Mitty HW, Rose J, et al: Ultrasonography of adrenal masses: Usual features. Radiology 127:467–474, 1978.
23. Gilday DL, Ash JM, Reilly BJ: Radionuclide skeletal survey for pediatric neoplasms. Radiology 123:399–406, 1977.
24. Barry JF, Harwood-Nash DC, Fitz CR, et al: Metrizamide in pediatric myelography. Radiology 124:409–418, 1977.
25. Lee BCP, Kazam E, Newman AD: Computed tomography of the spine and spinal cord. Radiology 128:95–102, 1978.
26. Freiberger RH: The role of the radiologist in the management of the child with a suspected bone tumor. Cancer 35:925–929, 1975.
27. Rosen G, Tan C, Sanmaneechai A, et al: The rationale for multiple drug chemotherapy in the treatment of osteogenic sarcoma. Cancer 35:936–945, 1975.
28. Suit HD: Role of therapeutic radiology in cancer of bone. Cancer 35:930–935, 1975.
29. Wilson JS, Korobkin M, Genant HK, Bovill EG: Computed tomography of musculoskeletal disorders. AJR 131:55–61, 1978.
30. Breiman RS, Castellino RA, Harrell GS, et al: Pathologic correlations in Hodgkin's disease and non-Hodgkin's lymphoma. Radiology 126:159–166, 1978.
31. Filly RA, Marglin S, Castellino RA: The spectrum of subdiaphragmatic Hodgkin's disease and non-Hodgkin's lymphoma. Cancer 38:2143–2148, 1976.
32. Pilepich MV, Rene JB, Munzenrider JE, et al: Contribution of computed tomography to the treatment of lymphomas. AJR 131:69–73, 1978.
33. Lee JKT, Stanley RJ, Sagel SS, et al: Accuracy of computed tomography in detecting intra-abdominal and pelvic adenopathy in lymphoma. AJR 131:311–315, 1978.
34. Levine PH, Cho BR, Connelly RR, et al: The American Burkitt Lymphoma Registry: A progress report. Ann Intern Med 83:31–36, 1976.
35. Donaldson SS, Castro JR, Wilbur JR, Jesse RH: Rhabdomyosarcoma of the head and neck in children: Combination treatment by surgery, irradiation, and chemotherapy. Cancer 31:26–35, 1973.

36. Ghavimi F, Exelby PR, D'Angio GJ, et al: Combination therapy of urogenital embryonal rhabdomyosarcoma in children. Cancer 32:1178–1185, 1973.
37. Weinstein MA, Levine H, Duchesneau PM, Tucker HM: Diagnosis of juvenile angiofibroma by computed tomography. Radiology 126:703–705, 1978.
38. Lawrence W Jr, Hays DM, Moon TE: Lymphatic metastasis with childhood rhabdomyosarcoma. Cancer 39:556–559, 1977.
39. Ambrose JAE, Lloyd GAS, Wright JE: A preliminary evaluation of fine matrix computerized axial tomography (EMI scan) in the diagnosis of orbital space-occupying lesions. Br J Radiol 47:747–751, 1974.

Index